T0100270

GENETICS – RESEARCH AND ISSUES

PHYLOGEOGRAPHY

CONCEPTS, INTRASPECIFIC PATTERNS AND SPECIATION PROCESSES

GENETICS – RESEARCH AND ISSUES

Additional books in this series can be found on Nova's website
under the Series tab.

Additional e-books in this series can be found on Nova's website
under the e-books tab.

GENETICS – RESEARCH AND ISSUES

PHYLOGEOGRAPHY

CONCEPTS, INTRASPECIFIC PATTERNS AND SPECIATION PROCESSES

DAMIEN S. RUTGERS
EDITOR

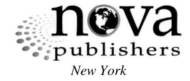

publishers
New York

NOTICE TO THE READER

The Publisher has taken reasonable care in the preparation of this book, but makes no expressed or implied warranty of any kind and assumes no responsibility for any errors or omissions. No liability is assumed for incidental or consequential damages in connection with or arising out of information contained in this book. The Publisher shall not be liable for any special, consequential, or exemplary damages resulting, in whole or in part, from the readers' use of, or reliance upon, this material. Any parts of this book based on government reports are so indicated and copyright is claimed for those parts to the extent applicable to compilations of such works.

Independent verification should be sought for any data, advice or recommendations contained in this book. In addition, no responsibility is assumed by the publisher for any injury and/or damage to persons or property arising from any methods, products, instructions, ideas or otherwise contained in this publication.

This publication is designed to provide accurate and authoritative information with regard to the subject matter covered herein. It is sold with the clear understanding that the Publisher is not engaged in rendering legal or any other professional services. If legal or any other expert assistance is required, the services of a competent person should be sought. FROM A DECLARATION OF PARTICIPANTS JOINTLY ADOPTED BY A COMMITTEE OF THE AMERICAN BAR ASSOCIATION AND A COMMITTEE OF PUBLISHERS.

Additional color graphics may be available in the e-book version of this book.

LIBRARY OF CONGRESS CATALOGING-IN-PUBLICATION DATA

Phylogeography : concepts, intraspecific patterns, and speciation processes
/ editors, Damien S. Rutgers.
      p. ; cm.
 Includes bibliographical references and index.
 ISBN: 978-1-60692-954-4 (hardcover)
 1. Phylogeography. 2. Population geography. I. Rutgers, Damien S.
 [DNLM: 1. Biological Phenomena. 2. Geography. 3. Genetic Variation. 4.
Genetics, Population. 5. Phylogeny. QH 84 P578 2010]
  QH84.P497 2010
  576.8'809--dc22
    2010007599

Published by Nova Science Publishers, Inc. † *New York*

CONTENTS

PREFACE

Phylogeography is the study of the historical processes that may be responsible for the contemporary geographic distributions of individuals. This is accomplished by considering the geographic distribution of individuals in light of the patterns associated with a gene genealogy. This term was introduced to describe geographically structured genetic signals within and among species. An explicit focus on a species' biogeography/biogeographical past sets phylogeography apart from classical population genetics and phylogenetics. This new book reviews research on phylogeography.

Chapter 1- Fishes constitute about half of all known vertebrate species and have colonized nearly all available marine and freshwater habitats. The greatest diversity of fishes is found in the marine realm as well as in large (and often old) freshwater lakes such as the East African Great Lakes. Here, the authors compare the phylogeographic history of fishes in marine and large freshwater ecosystems, with particular emphasis on groups that underwent adaptive radiation, *i.e.* the emergence of a multitude of species from a single ancestor as a consequence of the adaptation to different ecological niches. Phylogeographic analyses are highly suited to identify and compare causal agents of speciation in rapidly diversifying groups. This is particularly true for fishes, in which distribution ranges and preferred habitat structures can be quantified in a straightforward matter.

Chapter 2- Phylogeography involves knowledge of the spatial distribution of related individuals and historical information on the relationship within and among populations and species. The phylogeography of many groups has been studied over recent decades, and this field of knowledge is now becoming important in solving the problems of pest control in agriculture and forestry. An understanding of the nature of the genetic variation within and between pest populations is of paramount importance in the design of pest control programmes and their success – and successful programs are certainly needed since increasing levels of trade and passenger travel, the growth of new plant species in new regions and climate change are all assisting the spread of economically important insect pests. Molecular genetics is now providing us with new and more sensitive tools for developing appropriate insect control and eradication strategies. The author's group is studying the genetic variation of tephritids and whiteflies, both of which are important pests of agricultural and ornamental plants in the Mediterranean region (ecosystems). The information presented here is a summary of some of the results obtained in enzyme electrophoresis (MLEE), abundant soluble protein content, random amplification of polymorphic DNA (RAPD-PCR), intermicrosatellite (ISSR), restriction fragment length polymorphism (RFLP) and mtDNA sequencing analyses. These data document the phylogeographic structure of these taxa's populations, and provide information regarding their bioinvasion and colonisation of new areas, their geographic variation, and gene flow among regions. Such information could be helpful in the taking of pest management decisions, and highlights the need for the coordination of control programs between regional, national and international authorities.

Chapter 3- Parasitic plants have aroused curiosity among scientists for centuries, yet they remain one of the most poorly understood groups of flowering plants (angiosperms), and much of their evolutionary biology remains a mystery. There are approximately 4,000 species of parasitic plants (in 19 families) which occur in all major biomes, from arctic islands to tropical forests. The evolutionary shift to parasitism has been associated with the degeneration of morphological features traditionally used in plant classification to infer evolutionary relationships, making systematic studies of the relationships between parasitic plants and their photosynthetic ancestors extremely difficult. Therefore until very recently, the author's understanding of the evolutionary origins of parasitic angiosperms has lagged behind that of other major groups of angiosperms. Parasitic plants show considerable variation in their host specificity. For example, some species infect hundreds of species from taxonomically diverse families, while others are restricted to a single host species. Host ecology may isolate parasite populations and facilitate genetic divergence. For example in leaf-eating (phytophagus) insects which, like parasitic plants, are discriminate users with respect to the host plants on which they feed, host specificity has been demonstrated to drive genetic divergence, and ultimately speciation. However speciation in parasitic plants has, until recently, remained relatively unexplored by evolutionary biologists, and understanding of host specificity as a potential catalyst for speciation in these plants has lagged behind that of phytophagus insects. Now, in light of recent research, a similar pattern of host-driven speciation in parasitic plants is emerging. This chapter reviews recent research into the host specificity of parasitic plants, which appears to be an important and underestimated promoter of genetic divergence and speciation.

Chapter 4- Gene flow and genetic drift are important factors affecting geographic variation of human phenotypic traits. In the present study, the effects of gene flow from an outside source on the pattern of within- and among-group variation of Hokkaido Ainu, one of the most generalized eastern Asian populations, are examined by applying R-matrix method to 24 nonmetric cranial traits. The R-matrix method is developed initially for single-locus traits and modified for use with quantitative (metric) phenotypic data. In this study, tetrachoric correlation coefficients estimated by maximum likelihood method, the threshold value for each trait estimated by univariate probit analysis, and the census population sizes of the regional groups of the recent Ainu were used for applying the R-matrix method to nonmetric morphological data. Within-group variance based on nonmetric data was estimated by bootstrap sampling method. The results obtained suggest the possibility of admixture between the immigrants from Northeast Asia as represented by the Okhotsk culture people and the indigenous inhabitants in Hokkaido during the 5th – 12th centuries A.D., at least in the coastal region along the Sea of Okhotsk. Such gene flow from Northeast Asian continent may have a certain degree of effect on genetic structure of recent Ainu as suggested from morphological and ancient mitochondrial DNA evidence. The present findings suggest, moreover, a possible inter-population relationship between the Ainu and non-Ainu Japanese at recent period of time. The present analyses provide results that can be interpreted in terms of archaeologically and historically suggested pattern of gene flow and isolation.

Chapter 5- Phylogeography uses present day geographic patterns of genotypes to infer the historical distribution and demography of species. While species-specific patterns have been interesting, repeated geographic patterns across species, known as phylogeographic concordance, provide evidence for general mechanisms and biogeographic events that have together shaped the distribution and diversity of genotypes. As the evidence for phylogeographic concordance started to accumulate, phylogeographers began to revisit the concept of suture zones. Suture zones, as originally described by Charles Remington, are geographic regions where multiple sister species pairs experience secondary contact and hybridize. Of interest was that some of Remington's suture zones seemed to include regions of phylogeographic concordance, suggesting that the concept and mechanisms behind the formation of suture zones could be translated from hybrid zone research to phylogeographic research. Thus, the challenge now is to explore whether a full integration of the concepts of suture zone formation and phylogeographic concordance is possible and how the authors should test for their existence. Here author will discuss the suture zone concept and how it relates to phylogeographic concordance, discuss previous attempts to statistically test for the existence of suture zones and phylogeographic concordance, and propose a more rigorous statistical analytical approach towards testing for the existence of suture zones and phylogeographic concordance.

Chapter 6- The insular East Asia contains many islands encompasses various climatic regions, from subtropical to subarctic. Its fauna contains about 400 species of the order Odonata (dragonflies and damselflies), including many endemic ones. Two groups of dragonflies, the genus *Davidius* and *Anotogaster sieboldii* show interesting radiation patterns in this region. Both the mitochondrial and nuclear gene genealogy revealed that four species of the genus *Davidius* in this region seem to have diversified through the geographical connection and disconnection between the Korean Peninsula and Japanese main islands. The habitat of the larvae of *D. moiwanus* sspp. were estimated to have shifted from rivers to narrow streams in wetlands. Molecular phylogeographical analyses revealed not only their divergence history in the insular region but also including the process divided them from the continental congeners. Mitochondrial gene genealogy based on COI gene sequence data revealed that *A. sieboldii* includes two deeply differentiated clades that seem to have diverged in late Miocene or early Plicocene. Each of these two clades includes three inner clades that seem to have differentiated in Pleistocene.

Chapter 7- Recent statistical phylogeographic work has sought to integrate ecological niche models (ENMs) into phylogeography as a methodology for testing and formulating hypotheses regarding the geographic histories of species. The lure of ENMs lies in their ability to use present day climatic and physiographic affinities of species to predict the past geographic distributions of these same species under different climatic regimes. These predicted distributions can then be used to evaluate the likelihood and location of glacial refugia. Given the bourgeoning interest in ENMs, now is an appropriate time for phylogeographers to reexamine their conceptual and methodological foundations. The authors argue that in the rush to assimilate this methodology, critical underlying assumptions have not been adequately considered. Here the authors discuss some of the fundamental assumptions underlying ENMs and how their violation may lead to faulty phylogeographic inferences. The authors will conclude by discussing alternative avenues for future research that will enable a more reliable and fruitful integration of ENM and phylogeography.

Chapter 8- Phylogeography focuses on the study of the geographical structure of gene lineages within single species. The aim to analyze how phylogenetic relationships of genealogical lineages are distributed across the geographical landscape makes phylogeography a discipline embedded in the wider field of biogeography which is primarily concerned with inference and, possibly, identification of the major processes shaping organismal diversity at different levels of geographical and taxonomical scales. The adoption of molecular data to infer patterns of genetic variation interpreted in a geographical context positively affected biogeographical research: many fruitful insights can be gained about the different roles of bottlenecks, population expansions, vicariance and gene flow in structuring genetic variability. From its inception, at least two major breakthroughs occurred in phylogeography: the advent of comparative phylogeography and the use of model-based statistical analysis which led to statistical phylogeography. The comparative approach involves the comparison among co-distributed taxa of geographical patterns of genetic variation thus allowing detailed inferences to be drawn about, for instance, landscape evolution, dispersal across a region, speciation, extinction and adaptive radiation. Linking population processes to regional biogeographical and diversity patterns can have important outcomes also for ecology and evolution studies. Historically and evolutionary independent regions can be identified, statistically testing their independence through adequate state-of-art analytical methods. Determining the evolutionary and geographical framework, phlyogeography can shed light on the spatial and historical influences governing the distribution of species richness in ecological communities. Finally, the possibility to identify evolutionary isolated areas is of great importance as a tool to better design conservation strategies. The efforts to preserve and manage biodiversity can, therefore, greatly benefit from the results of comparative phylogeography by allowing understanding the processes responsible, both locally and a regional level, for origin, evolution, diversification and maintenance of communities. The advent of several coalescent-based analytical methods has somehow revolutionized the interpretation of genetic data; instead of simply describing the data in search of *ad hoc* explanations, it's now possible to statistically test whether the data fit some historical and demographic scenario. Several hypotheses about the processes underlying patterns of genetic variability and structure can now rigorously tested in a reasonable amount of computation time, thanks also to the technical improvement in computer technology. It is now widely recognized that further development of coalescent-based methods, also with extensive use of Bayesian approaches, can significantly contribute to phylogeography studies. Despite these premises, it seems that most of current phylogeographical literature is still centered around the analysis of a single genetic marker in a single species.

Chapter 9- *Fringillidae* finches form a subfamily of songbirds (*Passeriformes*), which are presently distributed around the world. This subfamily includes canaries, goldfinches, greenfinches, rosefinches, and grosbeaks, among others. Molecular phylogenies obtained with mitochondrial DNA sequences show that these groups of finches are put together, but with some polytomies that have apparently evolved or radiated in parallel. The time of appearance on Earth of all studied groups is suggested to start after Middle Miocene Epoch, around 10 million years ago. Greenfinches (genus *Carduelis*) may have originated at Eurasian desert margins coming from *Rhodopechys obsoleta* (dessert finch) or an extinct pale plumage ancestor; it later acquired green plumage suitable for the greenfinch ecological niche, i.e.: woods. Multicolored Eurasian goldfinch (*Carduelis carduelis*) has a genetic extant ancestor, the green-feathered *Carduelis citrinella* (citril finch); this was thought to be a canary on phonotypical bases, but it is now included within goldfinches by the author's molecular genetics phylograms. Speciation events between citril finch and Eurasian goldfinch are related with the Mediterranean Messinian salinity crisis (5 million years ago). *Linurgus olivaceus* (oriole finch) is presently thriving in Equatorial Africa and was included in a separate genus (*Linurgus*) by itself on phenotypical bases. The author's phylograms demonstrate that it is and old canary. Proposed genus *Acanthis* does not exist. Twite and linnet form a separate radiation from redpolls. *Loxia* (crossbills) is an evolutive radiation which includes redpolls also. In North America, three *Carduelis* radiations are found all coming from the Eurasian siskin: 1) that of American goldfinch, 2) the pine siskin one, and 3) the *Carduelis notata* one, ancestor of all South American siskins. A new group of 'arid-zone' finches is genetically described that includes *Leucosticte arctoa*, *Carpodacus nipalensis*, *Rhodopechys githaginea* and *Rhodopechys mongolica*, at least. Genus *Rhodopechys* should be redefined. *Pinicola enucleator* (pine grosbeak) is the ancestor of bullfinches (genus *Pyrrhula*), forming a single evolutive radiation. Genus *Carpodacus* has been split in several evolutive radiations; American *Carpodacus* form a distinct evolution from Old World *Carpodacus*. *Haematospiza sipahi* is not a single genus, but a radiation together with *Carpodacus erythrinus*. Another evolutive radiation is found: *Uragus sibiricus* (a single species genus) radiated together with *Carpodacus rubicilloides*. The grosbeak radiation (*Emberizinae*) occurred earlier than that of other *Fringillidae* birds and comprises genera *Coccothraustes*, *Eophona*, and *Mycerobas*. It is not discarded that New World grosbeaks (*Hesperiphona*) is also related. Old World sparrows (genus *Passer*) conforms a single radiation starting in Africa (with *P. melanurus* and grey-headed sparrows), separated from *Ploceinae* and New and Old World *Emberizinae*. The closest radiation to genus *Passer* is genus *Petronia* (rock sparrows). *Passer hispaniolensis italiae* (brown head) is genetically closer to *P. domesticus* (grey head) than to *P. hispaniolensis* (brown head). Subfamily Estrildinae cover a variety of finches widespread through Africa, Asia, Australia, and Indian and Pacific Ocean islands. Yet, many evolutive radiations are observed within this monophyletic group; they comprise birds from different continents: genetics does not correlate with geography in these birds. A possible origin for them is India since the basal and most ancient evolutive radiation —comprising African silverbill, Indian silverbill and (Australian) diamond firetail— may have started in India. A clear example of convergent evolution is the case of American Carduelis dominicensis and African Linurgus olivaceus, which are very similar and acquire black head and greenish / yellow plumage in equatorial forests. Another fine example of phenotypic adaptation to environment is that of Serinus alario, the one black and white canary, because it nests on land or land / rocks. Finally, Eurasian goldfinch ancestor, mainly-green Carduelis citrinella, shows how plumage can change in relatively short times, as postulated. In summary, some examples of evolution details and misclassification of songbirds are shown and put in a paleoclimatic and geographical context. This is now possible because of the existence of powerful computation methodologies for constructing molecular phylogenetic trees which are changing both the view of evolution and classification of living beings.

In: Phylogeography   ISBN: 978-1-60692-954-4
Editor: Damien S. Rutgers   © 2013 Nova Science Publishers, Inc.

Chapter 1

PHYLOGEOGRAPHY AND SPECIATION PROCESSES IN MARINE FISHES AND FISHES FROM LARGE FRESHWATER LAKES

Michael Matschiner[1], Reinhold Hanel[2]*
and Walter Salzburger[1]

[1]Zoological Institute, University of Basel, Basel, Switzerland
[2]Institute of Fisheries Ecology, Johann Heinrich von Thünen-Institute,
Hamburg, Germany

ABSTRACT

Fishes constitute about half of all known vertebrate species and have colonized nearly all available marine and freshwater habitats. The greatest diversity of fishes is found in the marine realm as well as in large (and often old) freshwater lakes such as the East African Great Lakes. Here, we compare the phylogeographic history of fishes in marine and large freshwater ecosystems, with particular emphasis on groups that underwent adaptive radiation, *i.e.* the emergence of a multitude of species from a single ancestor as a consequence of the adaptation to different ecological niches. Phylogeographic analyses are highly suited to identify and compare causal agents of speciation in rapidly diversifying groups. This is particularly true for fishes, in which distribution ranges and preferred habitat structures can be quantified in a straightforward matter.

Keywords: adaptive radiation, gene flow, cichlids, notothenioids, labrids

* Author of correspondence.Reinhold Hanel
E-mail: reinhold.hanel@vti.bund.de

PHYLOGEOGRAPHY OF FISHES IN LARGE WATER BODIES

Since Avise *et al.* (1987) first coined the term phylogeography 23 years ago, the field has burgeoned and matured, and became a viable discipline at the intersection of population genetics, phylogenetics and biogeography (Avise 1998; 2009). The field's main concern are the principles and processes that led to contemporary geographic distributions within and between closely related species (Avise 2000). Linking micro- and macroevolutionary approaches, phylogeography has contributed greatly to species conservation, ecology and evolutionary biology. It has been integrated into the concept of 'evolutionary significant unit' (ESU) that classifies distinct populations that merit separate management and are of high priority for conservation (Ryder 1986; Moritz 1994; Crandall *et al.* 2000). Phylogeography has documented the impact of historical events on extant fauna and flora in many instances, and notably so in the case of European Pleistocene glaciations that have shaped the distribution of a wide range of European taxa (see *e.g.* Taberlet *et al.* 1998; Salzburger *et al.* 2003; Debes et al. 2008). It has also provided insights into the process of speciation (Avise 2000) when, for example the spatial simplicity and temporal certainty of volcanic archipelagos like Hawaii and the Canaries allow reconstruction of sequence and timing of speciation events (Shaw *et al.* 1996; Juan *et al.* 1998; Nepokroeff *et al.* 2003; Dimitrov *et al.* 2008; Sequeira *et al.* 2008).

A sizeable body of phylogeographic literature comes from studies conducted on teleost fishes. To some extent, this has been motivated by interest in sustained fisheries management that relies on the conservation of genetic diversity in the targeted species (Bernatchez & Wilson 1998). But fishes have also proven to be particularly informative for phylogeographic investigations. Riverine and especially lacustrine fishes inhabit island-like environments that are analoguous to volcanic archipelagos in respect of datability and spatial arrangement, and thus are similarly suitable for speciation research (Salzburger *et al.* 2005). On the other hand, marine fishes are traditionally characterized by their great diversity, their continuous and temporally stable habitat, large-scale distribution ranges, and high potential for dispersal (Palumbi 1994). Despite these differences, phylogeographic studies of marine fish species yielded important insights into population structures and their causes, the origin of marine diversity and the impact of historic events (Muss *et al.* 2001; Lourie & Vincent 2004; Rocha *et al.* 2007; Rocha *et al.* 2008). It has been shown that Pleistocene glaciations left their mark even in tropical marine settings (due to lowered sea levels; Lourie & Vincent 2004) and the phylogeography of marine species occurring on both sides of the Isthmus of Panama highlights the impact of plate tectonics on speciation over longer time scales (reviewed by Lessios 1998). Similarly, recolonization of the Mediterranean following the reopening of the Straight of Gibraltar 5.2 million years ago (MYA) (Hsü *et al.* 1973; 1977) led to a multitude of cladogenesis events that could be recovered by means of phylogeography (Carreras-Carbonell *et al.* 2005; Paternello *et al.* 2007). Furthermore, comparative phylogeography provides an adequate tool to resolve the relative impact of the many distinct life histories of marine fishes to the distributions of populations and species (Dawson *et al.* 2006). The physical setting of marine habitats also allows conclusions about these traits to be corroborated by incorporation of oceanographic data into phylogeographic analyses, *e.g.* by comparison of gene flow estimates and current speeds (Matschiner *et al.* 2009).

Thus, riverine, lacustrine, as well as marine fishes provide valuable systems for phylogeographic studies. Here, we compare the phylogeographic history of and patterns of speciation in fishes in marine and large freshwater ecosystems, with particular emphasis on groups that underwent adaptive radiation. We also present a literature review, in which we map the geographic patterns of gene flow in fish species from various taxonomic groups living in diverse environments.

The (Phylo-) Geography of Speciation

One of the most hotly debated questions in speciation is certainly its geography, and, in particular, whether geographic isolation is required for new biological entities to emerge (Coyne & Orr 2004; Gavrilets 2004). Clearly, speciation can only occur via the evolution of reproductive isolation between diverging lineages. For a long time allopatric speciation[1] has been advanced as major – or even exclusive – mode of speciation (Mayr 1942; Mayr 1963). This is somewhat surprising, given that Darwin himself considered all three modes of speciation plausible (see *e.g.* Coyne & Orr 2004): allopatric[1], sympatric[2], and parapatric[3]. Since sympatric and parapatric speciation has been backed-up with theoretical and empirical evidence over the last two decades (Schliewen *et al.* 1994; Dieckmann & Doebeli 1999; Higashi *et al.* 1999; Kondrashov & Kondrashov 1999; Barluenga *et al.* 2006; Gavrilets *et al.* 2007), the debate has now shifted towards the relative importance of each of these three modes of speciation in nature.

The three possible modes of speciation explicitly impart information about geography, individual migration and gene flow. In allopatric speciation, there is absolutely no migration of individuals between the (isolated) geographic areas occupied by the speciating sub-populations; no gene flow is possible. In sympatric speciation, there is but one place, and all individuals of the speciating entities live there. Thus, there is maximum migration of individuals between the (overlapping) distribution ranges of the diverging sub-populations. This does not mean, however, that individuals belonging to distinct entities interbreed (they may do so occasionally). It simply means that individuals migrate freely in space. In parapatric speciation, a certain degree of migration occurs between the distribution ranges of the speciating sub-populations (Gavrilets 2004), and in this case interbreeding and hybrid zones are an inert feature (see *e.g.* Wu 2001; Gavrilets 2004).

There is thus an obvious and strong link between the study of speciation and phylogeography: Phylogeography provides the concepts and tools to characterize past and ongoing gene flow – and, hence, migration – in the context of geography (see *e.g.* Avise 2009). Intentionally or not intentionally, most speciation research has thus relied on and greatly benefited from phylogeography. And whenever it is necessary to explicitly interlink gene flow and distribution range – for example when testing for sympatric speciation –

---

[1] *Allopatric speciation* describes the situation that there is complete geographic isolation between the speciating entities.

[2] *Sympatric speciation* can best be defined as the emergence of novel species from a population in which mating is random with respect to the birthplace of the mating partners (Gavrilets 2004).

[3] *Parapatric speciation* is everything in between complete geographic isolation and, hence, no migration between the diverging populations (allopatry) and full sympatry; it can also be described as speciation with gene flow (Wu 2001).

phylogeography is the best way to do so (see *e.g.* Barluenga *et al.* 2006; Savolainen *et al.* 2006).

Marine *versus* Lacustrine Adaptive Radiations in Fishes

Adaptive radiation is a process in which many species evolve in a short period of time by either allopatric, sympatric or parapatric speciation. It is the rapid proliferation of an ecologically and morphologically differentiated species assemblage from one ancestral species as a consequence of the adaptation to various ecological niches (Schluter 2000) – a process that is thought to have shaped much of the diversity of life. According to Schluter (2000), adaptive radiations can be detected by four main criteria: (*i*) common ancestry of the diversifying clade; (*ii*) a correlation between morphological or physiological traits of divergent lineages and their respective environments; (*iii*) evidence for the actual utility of these traits in their environments; and (*iv*) the rapid evolution of reproductive isolation between individuals of the divergent lineages. Often – but not always – adaptive radiations occur after the colonization of a new habitat or the evolution of evolutionary 'key innovations' (Gavrilets & Vose 2005). As a consequence of the rapid cladogenesis at the onset of an adaptive radiation, phylogenies of the radiating groups are typically bottom-heavy (Gavrilets & Vose 2005) and non-bifurcating (Sturmbauer *et al.* 2003). There are not many adaptive radiations, though, for which the fulfillment of all four criteria and bottom-heavy phylogenies has been fully demonstrated.

The most famous textbook examples of adaptive radiations are the Darwin's finches on the Galapagos archipelago (see *e.g.* Grant & Grant 2002; Grant & Grant 2006), the Caribbean *Anoles* lizards (see *e.g.* Losos *et al.* 1998), and the species flocks of cichlid fishes in the Great Lakes of East Africa (Box 1). With an estimated number of at least 1,500 species, the assemblages of cichlid fishes in lakes Victoria, Malawi and Tanganyika constitute the most diverse and species-rich adaptive radiations known (Seehausen 2006; Salzburger 2009). There are, however, at least 20 more lacustrine adaptive radiations in cichlids in Africa (Seehausen 2006); and cichlid adaptive radiations are also known from outside the African continent, *e.g.*, in the Great Lakes of Nicaragua and some smaller crater lakes nearby (Barluenga & Meyer 2004; Barluenga *et al.* 2006). Why cichlid fishes are obviously prone for adaptive radiation and explosive speciation is still under debate. It seems plausible, though, that their evolutionary success rests on a unique interaction of external factors such as habitat structure and ecological opportunity and intrinsic characteristics in form of life-history traits and evolutionary key innovations like a highly adaptable feeding apparatus (Salzburger 2009).

Adaptive radiations in teleost fishes are, in general, quite common in freshwater systems: Three-spined sticklebacks (*Gasterosteus aculeatus*), for example, have repeatedly radiated into benthic and limnetic forms from ancestral marine ecotypes in post-glacial lakes (Schluter & McPhail 1992); lake whitefish (*Coregonus* spp.) have undergone adaptive radiations in post-glacial lakes, too, throughout their distribution range in the Northern hemisphere (Bernatchez *et al.* 1999; Ostbye *et al.* 2005; Vonlanthen *et al.* 2009); in the Malili lake system in Sulawesi, several species of sailfin silversides (*Telmatherina* spp.) have emerged via adaptive radiation (Herder *et al.* 2006; Roy *et al.* 2007a; Roy *et al.* 2007b); adaptive radiations have also been proposed in African weakly electric fish (*Campylomormyrus* spp.) (Feulner *et al.* 2007), in barbs (*Labeobarbus* spp.) from Lake Tana in Ethiopia (de Graaf *et al.* 2008), in cyprinids from Philippine Lake Lanao (Kornfield & Carpenter 1984), and in cyprinodontids (*Orestias* spp.) from Lake Titicaca in South America (Parenti 1984).

The situation is different in the marine realm, where much fewer cases of adaptive radiations have been described (see *e.g.* Rüber & Zardoya 2005). One group that fulfills all four criteria of an adaptive radiation are the notothenioid fishes that are mainly found in Antarctic waters (Eastman 2005) (Box 2). Several evolutionary key-innovations and adaptiations have been identified (in notothenioids and subgroups thereof) that allow them to cope with the harsh environmental conditions in the Southern Ocean, such as the evolution of antifreeze glycoproteins and the losses of hemoglobin, of parts of the mitochondrial respiratory chain and of the heat-shock response system (Chen *et al.* 1997; di Prisco *et al.* 2002; Papetti *et al.* 2007a; Hofmann *et al.* 2000). However, the radiation of the whole Antarctic clade does not exhibit the bottom-heavy phylogeny (*sensu* Gavrilets & Vose 2005) theoretically expected in adaptive radiations. Instead, the full notothenioid species richness of about 130 species is attained through at least three secondary radiations – those of the artedidraconid genus *Pogonophryne*, the nototheniid subfamily *Trematominae* and the nototheniid genus *Patagonotothen* (Eastman 2005; Sanchez *et al.* 2007; Near & Cheng 2008).

Other radiations in marine fishes are less well documented than the notothenioid one and it remains to be proven whether some of these radiations are 'adaptive' after all. A second teleost radiation may have occurred in the Antarctic region. The deeper parts of the Antarctic shelf are inhabited by 64 species of the scorpaeniform family Liparidae that probably represent a secondary radiation within a larger liparid diversification, centered mainly in the North Pacific region (Eastman & Clarke 1998). The colorful parrotfishes (Scaridae), unambiguously shown to be a specialized lineage deeply nested within the family Labridae (Bellwood 1994, Westneat & Alfaro 2005), inhabit the coral reefs and seagrass beds of tropical waters. Its roughly 90 species have adapted to a variety of habitats as well as social and mating strategies in the course of a radiation that presumably started around 14 MYA in the Tethys Sea (Streelman *et al.* 2002). The overall about 600 labrid species might as well represent an adaptive radiation (Box 3), and it has been argued that – just as in cichlid fishes – a highly adaptable pharyngeal jaw apparatus might have contributed as evolutionary key innovation in that group triggering their radiation (Westneat & Alfaro 2005; Mabuchi *et al.* 2007). Reef-associated gobies, such as the American seven-spined gobies (Gobioseomatini) or the Neotropical reef gobies (*Elacatinus* spp.) apparently underwent adaptive radiations, too (Rüber *et al.* 2003; Taylor & Hellberg 2005). Recently, Puebla and coworkers (Puebla *et al.* 2007; Puebla *et al.* 2008) have highlighted an example of a marine adaptive radiation in its very first stages, once again in colorful coral reef fishes, the hamlets (genus *Hypoplectrus*, family Serranidae). These 13 closely related predatory fish species are widely distributed in the Caribbean Sea.

It is not entirely obvious why adaptive radiation should be less frequent in marine fishes compared to those in (large) freshwater lakes. One reason why there are fewer cases reported in marine fishes might be that adaptive radiations are simply more apparent in geologically young and geographically well-defined areas (Salzburger 2008), and, hence, more easy to investigate. Indeed, the best candidates for adaptive radiations in marine fishes occurred in geographically separated areas such as the Antarctic continent (notothenioids) or the Caribbean Sea (hamlets). Older radiations, especially in tropical marine perciform families like wrasses, damselfishes, butterflyfishes, angelfishes as well as seabreams and others, date back much longer in time and might also be camouflaged by subsequent geographical separation through climatically and geologically induced range shifts or local extinctions.

THE GEOGRAPHIC SCALE OF GENE FLOW IN FISHES

Because of several reasons, fishes are an ideal group for phylogeographic research: their living space is strictly bordered by migration barriers (*e.g.* land, waterfalls, open water), their habitats are relatively easy to characterize, migration can only follow certain routes (*e.g.* ocean currents, coastlines, rivers), life-history traits (*e.g.* vagility, generation time, number of offspring) are often known, genetic tools are available, *etc.* Thus, it does not come to any surprise that a whole body of literature exists with respect to the phylogeography of various species of fish. For similar reasons, fishes are excellent models for speciation and adaptive radiation research (see *e.g.* Kocher 2004; Rüber & Zardoya 2005; Seehausen 2006; Rocha & Bowen 2008; Salzburger 2009).

Migration, gene flow and genetic differentiation are crucial parameters in both phylogeography and speciation (see above). In order to compare geographic distances over which genetic differentiation takes place in different environments and different groups of fishes, we conducted a literature review and focused on phylogeographic and population genetic studies according to the following criteria: (*i*) either DNA sequences or microsatellite loci were used as molecular markers, (*ii*) sample sizes and sampling locations were specified precisely, (*iii*) pairwise *F*-statistics or similar measures were reported, (*iv*) sequential Bonferroni correction for multiple tests (Rice 1989) or a false discovery rate (Benjamini & Hochberg 1995) was applied to pairwise comparisons, or *p*-values were reported and enabled us to conduct Bonferroni error correction. We ignored studies on populations of unresolved species status, and those that include artificially introduced or cultured populations, as well as studies investigating populations separated by artificial barriers such as river dams. Riverine populations were included only if they were sampled from the same watershed. For every study, we measured both the shortest water connection over which significant genetic differentiation was found (d_{min_s}) and the longest water connection over which no significant gene flow could be detected (d_{max_ns}). All geographic distances were measured using Google Earth®. Exact sampling locations were rarely given for anadromous species from different river systems. In these cases, the distance between river estuaries was taken. We particularly focused on three groups of perciform fishes that underwent adaptive radiations in three distinct environments: cichlids (lacustrine), labrids (tropical to temperate marine), and notothenioids (polar marine).

We based our comparison on 81 articles (marked with * in the References) investigating the population genetic stucture of 114 fish species in environments as diverse as the Arctic and the Great Barrier Reef, the Amazon River and the 34 km long Atsuta River in Japan. A number of species was investigated in more than one study or with both nucleotide and microsatellite markers, so that we ended up with 130 measurements of d_{min_s} and/or d_{max_ns}. In 37 cases, no significant genetic differentiation was found between investigated populations, while all pairwise comparisons were significant in 25 out of the 130 cases. In the most extreme cases, significant genetic differentiation was found between samples taken at the same location, but in different years (d_{min_s} = 0 km; Zane *et al.* 2006; Lin *et al.* 2008a; Hepburn *et al.* 2009), or no comparison was significant despite a global sampling scheme (d_{max_ns} = 16,309 km; Horne *et al.* 2008).

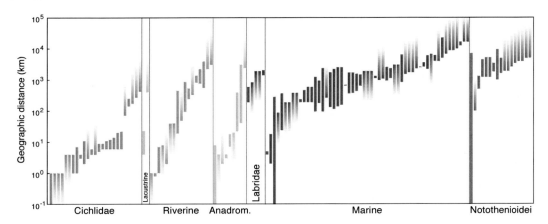

Figure 1. The geographic scale of gene flow in fishes. Shortest geographic distances over which significant genetic population differentiation have been found in different taxonomic groups and environments. Each bar represents one analysis of population differentiation. Bars are drawn between the shortest distance, over which significant differentiation has been found (d_{min_s}), and the longest distance, over which no significant differentiation could be detected (d_{max_ns}). A downward gradient symbolizes that all pairwise comparisons were significant. In these cases, the gradient's top end represents d_{min_s}. This visualizes that significant differentiation could be expected at even shorter, untested distances. Similarly, an upward gradient symbolizes that no pairwise comparison was significant, and that significant differentiation can be expected only at distances greater than those tested (d_{max_ns} is the gradients lower end). All distances were measured as the shortest water connections between fish populations.

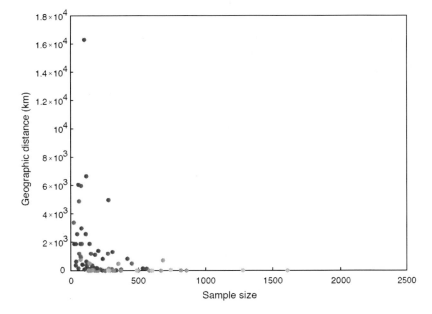

Figure 2. Sample size effects in phylogeographic studies in fishes. The shortest geographic distance over which significant differentiation has been detected plotted against sample size. Color code as in Figure 1.

The shortest geographic distances, over which significant genetic differentiation was found in different taxonomic groups and environments are visualized in Figure 1. Naturally, these measures may depend on parameters such as study design, sample size and number of markers employed. In Figure 2, we plotted d_{min_s} against the sample size of the respective study. Indeed, the result suggests a negative correlation between both values. However, as the average sample sizes were comparable between studies in different fish taxa and environments (with the exception of anadromous fishes: N = 825; others: N = 130-333), the overall picture shown in Figure 1 should not be influenced by the different study practices applied by the different researcher groups.

Lacustrine Fishes

Differentiation over short geographic distances on the order of 10 km and below is commonly found in rock-dwelling cichlids of the East African Great Lakes, and it has been speculated whether their tendency to philopatry and the resulting barriers to gene flow has enabled local adaptation, speciation, and their impressive adaptive radiation (Rico & Turner 2002; Pereyra *et al.* 2004). However, the cichlid radiations also include a number of pelagic species that show genetic homogeneity over hundreds of kilometers, and thus would contradict this hypothesis (see the five bars at the right end of the Cichlidae column in Fig. 1) (Shaw *et al.* 2000; Taylor & Verheyen 2001). We found two studies on non-cichlid lacustrine fishes that matched our criteria: Sailfin silversides of Lake Matano, Indonesia, show significant differentiation at small geographic distances (Walter *et al.* 2009), while large-scale gene flow was observed in the little Baikal oilfish in Lake Baikal, Russia (Teterina *et al.* 2005).

Riverine and Anadromous Fishes

Very variable patterns were found in riverine and anadromous fish species. In the case of the riverine fishes, it appears that river size influences rates of gene flow between populations: Genetic differentiation over short distances was found repeatedly in small river systems such as the Caroni Drainage, Trinidad and Tobago (d_{min_s} = 1 km, all comparisons being significant; Barson *et al.* 2009), the Amor de Cosmos watershed on Vancouver Island, Canada (d_{min_s}, d_{max_ns} = 1 km; Caldera & Bolnick 2008), and the Novoselka River basin, Sakhalin, Russia (d_{min_s} = 1 km, d_{max_ns} = 7 km; Osinov & Gordeeva 2008). On the other hand, population genetic assessments of fishes of the Amazon River frequently fail to detect significant population structure over the entire sampling area (d_{max_ns} > 2000 km; Batista & Alves-Gomes 2006; Santos *et al.* 2007).

Marine Fishes

In general, marine fishes show great variability in their patterns of differentiation: While reef fishes with low dispersal abilities may exhibit significant population structure at less than 10 km (Miller-Sims *et al.* 2008; Bay *et al.* 2008), most marine fishes display differentiation only at distances of hundreds to thousands of kilometers; no genetic structuring even at a global scale has been observed in lemon sharks (Schultz *et al.* 2008) and two surgeonfishes (Horne *et al.* 2008). Fishes of the family Labridae show comparable patterns of differentiation between the different species. Significant population structure was found between 187 and 1898 km. Fishes of the perciform suborder Notothenioidei show little genetic structuring even compared to other marine fish taxa. One exception aside (significant structure between year-classes sampled at the same location; Zane *et al.* 2006), significant genetic differentiation has been found only over several hundreds or thousands of kilometers, or not at all, as is the case for the majority of studies included in our survey. As the life histories of most notothenioids include long pelagic larval stages of up to one and a half years (Kock & Kellermann 1991; La Mesa & Ashford 2008), it has been speculated that strong oceanic currents, and in particular the Antarctic Circumpolar Current (ACC) may be responsible for gene flow in form of larval dispersal (Zane *et al.* 2006; Jones *et al.* 2008). Using a multidisciplinary approach including oceanographic data and simulations using the isolation-with-migration (IM) model (Hey & Nielsen 2007) to investigate directionality of gene flow in the notothenioid fish *Gobionotothen gibberifrons*, Matschiner *et al.* (2009) indeed found highly asymmetric migration rates between the Antarctic Peninsula and islands of the Scotia Ridge, following the direction of the ACC. As gene flow caused by long-distance migration of adult individuals would be expected to result in roughly symmetric migration rates, this finding corroborates the hypothesis that larval dispersal precludes genetic differentiation in Antarctic waters even across large geographic distances.

THREE ADAPTIVELY RADIATING PERCIFORM GROUPS

At least one in two vertebrate species is a fish and within the fishes at least one third (and more than 10,000 species) belongs to the order Perciformes, making it the largest order of vertebrates. The Perciformes itself is comprised of about 160 families and more than 1500 genera and they dominate vertebrate life in the ocean and in tropical and subtropical freshwaters (Nelson 2006). Much of the diversity of perciforms has arisen through adaptive radiations, of which the ones of the cichlid fishes are the most impressive. Marine (adaptive) radiations within the Perciformes are those of the notothenioids, of the labrids, the gobies, and the hamlets (Eastman 2005; Westneat & Alfaro 2005; Rüber *et al.* 2003; Puebla *et al.* 2008). Massive bursts of diversification ('explosive speciation') have repeatedly been reported for East African cichlid fishes (*e.g.* McCune 1997; Seehausen 2002; Verheyen *et al.* 2003). In marine fishes, elevated rates of cladogenesis were reported – among others – for *Sebastes* rockfishes, the notothenioid subfamily Trematominae, American seven-spined gobies and sparids (Rüber & Zardoya 2005).

Here, we focus on three groups of Perciformes that apparently underwent adaptive radiations and episodes of explosive speciation in different environments (Eastman & Clarke 1998; Eastman 2005; Seehausen 2006; Mabuchi *et al.* 2007): the cichlids of the tropical Great Lakes in East Africa (Box 1), the notothenioids of the polar marine waters of Antarctica (Box 2), and the labrids of the tropical and subtropical marine waters (Box 3). The adaptive radiations of all three groups have been associated with evolutionary key-innovations (Liem 1973; Chen *et al.* 1997; Hulsey 2006; Mabuchi *et al.* 2007), they all evolved a spectacular diversity of body morphologies and – in the case of cichlids and labrids – color morphs, and members of all three groups dominate their respective fauna.

Phylogeographic and population genetic studies in the three groups cichlids, notothenioids, and labrids reveal substantial differences with respect to the geographic distances over which gene flow could be detected (Figure 1). While in most cichlid species population structure could be detected over small geographic ranges of below or around 10 km, labrids and – with one exception – notothenioids show gene flow over large geographic distances. The latter two groups lie well in the range of other marine fishes, just as a few pelagic cichlid species do (note that the upper geographic limits in these cichlid species is restricted by lake size). This discrepancy between gene flow on a circumantarctic scale in notothenioids and large distances in labrids and the fine-scale genetic structuring in cichlids of the East African Lakes seems puzzling, given that all these clades underwent adaptive radiations in their respective environments, and philopatry has often been proposed as one of the key agents behind local adaptation and, consequently, adaptive radiation (Bouton *et al.* 1999; Rico & Turner 2002; Rico *et al.* 2003; Pereyra *et al.* 2004; Taylor & Hellberg 2005; Gavrilets *et al.* 2007).

Gene flow is generally expected to retard speciation by breaking linkage between genes for local adaptation and those for reproductive isolation (Coyne & Orr 2004). On the other hand, recent theoretical work as well as empirical research (Gavrilets & Vose 2005; Seehausen 2006; Garant *et al.* 2007) has shown that gene flow between populations does not necessarily prevent local adaptation. To the contrary, it can facilitate the spread of beneficial mutations and thus support adaptation under certain circumstances. In the context of adaptive radiation, the individual-based stochastic model of Gavrilets & Vose (2005) predicted that divergence can be maintained for very long periods despite substantial amounts of gene flow, which would lead to a 'porous' genome with low to non-existing differentiation in neutral markers, but divergence at locally selected loci. Evidence for porous genomes has been found in the *Hypoplectrus* complex of coral reef fishes that are supposed to represent an adaptive radiation in its very first stages (Puebla *et al.* 2008).

PHYLOGEOGRAPHY AND SPECIATION IN MARINE *VERSUS* LACUSTRINE FISHES

So what is it that could explain the difference between marine fishes with gene flow over large geographic distances and fishes from large freshwater lakes with often highly structured populations?

Habitat discontinuities, which have been suggested as main reason why rock-dwelling cichlid populations are so structured (Arnegard *et al.* 1999; Rico & Turner 2002; Pereyra *et al.* 2004; Duftner *et al.* 2006; Sefc *et al.* 2007), can only partly explain these differences. Marine reefs are highly fragmented, too. Still, gene flow in reef associated fishes can be observed over large geographic distances, *e.g.* between the West and East Atlantic (Floeter *et al.* 2008; Rocha *et al.* 2008) or between Caribbean islands over hundreds of kilometers (Puebla *et al.* 2008). Habitats of benthic notothenioids are disrupted by iceberg scours (Brenner *et al.* 2001) and open water between island shelves, while the habitat of a limited number of pelagic notothenioids may be assumed continuous over thousands of kilometers

(Zane *et al.* 2006). Nevertheless, pelagic and benthic notothenioids alike apparently maintain gene flow over these large distances (Figure 1) (Matschiner *et al.* 2009).

Another extrinsic factor that might explain the observed differences in population structure is *habitat stability*. Large freshwater lakes are very young compared to marine habitats. Lake Tanganyika, for example, the oldest of the East African Great Lakes and second oldest lake in the world, has a maximum age of 12 million years (MY) (Cohen *et al.* 1997); Lakes Malawi and Victoria are considerably younger. More importantly, the lakes have repeatedly undergone dramatic water-level fluctuations of up to several hundred meters. In the case of Lake Victoria, this is equivalent to a complete desiccation, but fish diversity may have survived in tributaries and satellite lakes (Johnson *et al.* 1996; Cohen *et al.* 1997; Mwanja *et al.* 2001; Verheyen *et al.* 2003; Stager & Johnson 2008). It has been argued that these cyclic changes leading to admixis, hybridization, fragmentation of populations, and small founder populations, contributed to the species-richness in the East African lakes (Rossiter 1995; Kornfield & Smith 2000; Sturmbauer *et al.* 2001). It is less apparent, though, how these lake-level fluctuations could account for the structuring in present cichlid populations. Dramatic changes in the environment also characterize the marine habitat of Antarctic notothenioids. During the last two MY, the Antarctic ice sheet has periodically advanced and retreated with each glacial cycle. Presumably it has extended all the way to the shelf edge in glacial maxima (Thatje *et al.* 2005), 'bulldozing the surviving fauna to the deep continental margin' (Barnes & Conlan 2007). Naturally, the associated loss of benthic habitat must place serious constraints on demersal fish communities. There is evidence for at least some refuges in form of ice-free shelf areas (Barnes & Conlan 2007) that could provide analogues to satellite lakes of Lake Victoria during desiccation periods.

The temporal scale of significant and drastic environmental change is clearly different for wrasses and other tropical marine reef fishes and reaches back as far as the Eocene. The split of the most species-rich wrasse lineage, the Julidini, covering about one-third of overall labrid diversity was recently calculated of an age of 36 to 38 MY (Kazancioglu *et al.* 2009) supporting the hypothesis of their Tethyan origin and Indo-Pacific ancestral distribution (Westneat & Alfaro 2005). These estimates imply that by the time the julidine lineage originated, the Antarctic Circumpolar Current was already established, which disrupted the connection between higher and lower latitudes, and restricted the movement of tropical lineages to the Tethys (Bellwood & Wainwright 2002). A series of diversification events within the Julidini leading to an early burst of diversification and the evolution of the majority of extant julidine lineages nicely coincides with a period of increased diversification and fragmentation of coral reefs, and extensive development of reef communities in the Tethys and the Caribbean (Veron 1995) between 15 to 30 MY (Kazancioglu *et al.* 2009). Habitat fragmentation culminated in the middle Miocene with its rapidly changing paleobiogeographical conditions and strong tectonic activity (Rögl, 1999) that resulted in the final closure of seaway between the Mediterranean and the Indian Ocean some 14 MYA. Hanel *et al.* (2002) correlated the following succession of the Mediterranean with the radiation of the wrasse tribe Labrini, endemic to the northern Atlantic and found striking congruence.

Among the intrinsic (biotic) differences between marine fishes and fishes from large freshwater lakes is the *degree of specialization*. While most lacustrine East African cichlid species are ecologically highly specialized, the majority of marine fishes are not (at least not to the degree observed in cichlids). Rocha & Bowen (2008) attest that most reef fishes are 'neither widely distributed generalists nor ecological specialists'. Clearly, specialization limits gene flow by lowering survival rates and reproductive success of migrants. The question remains whether the much greater degree of specialization is a reason for or the outcome of the limited levels of gene flow between cichlid populations.

Another difference between marine fishes and cichlids is the *breeding behavior*. It is interesting though that in all three groups that underwent adaptive radiations, cichlids, notothenioids and labrids, a certain degree of brood care occurs. The cichlids are famous for their various systems and strategies of brood care behavior ranging from substrate spawning in nests and under custody of the parents to various levels of mouthbrooding (Goodwin *et al.* 1998; Barlow 2000).

Prolonged incubation and pelagic larval duration are common features of most Antarctic notothenioids (Kock & Kellermann 1991, Loeb *et al.* 1993). For example, hatching of larvae of the naked dragonfish *Gymnodraco acuticeps* occurs only about 10 months post-fertilization (Evans *et al.* 2005), while the Scotia Sea icefish *Chaenocephalus aceratus* undergoes an extensive pelagic phase as long as 1.5 years (La Mesa & Ashford 2008). Brood care of demersal eggs has been reported for a number of species and even egg carrying behavior has been observed in one icefish species (*Chionobathyscus dewitti*; Kock *et al.* 2006). However, other nototheniod fishes are open spawners that release their eggs in the open water column, or produce demersal eggs that become pelagic towards the end of their development (Kock 2005; Kellermann 1991). Pelagic eggs and larvae are prone to off-shelf advection and dispersal with strong oceanic currents such as the ACC. While active larval behavior, especially towards the end of the larval phase, may counteract dispersal in many cases (White 1998; Leis 2006), pelagic eggs and larvae have been found hundreds of kilometers away from suitable shelf habitat (Kellermann 1991; Loeb *et al.* 1993). Widespread larval dispersal is further suggested by the fact that only nototheniids and channichthyids with particularly long pelagic larval durations occur at the isolated island of Bouvetøya (Jones *et al.* 2008).

Within the percomorpha, the family Labridae can be considered exceptional in terms of diversity of social and reproductive systems. Most wrasses are sequential hermaphrodites, with a transformation from female to male state being the normal occurrence. The causes and pathways of the evolution of hermphroditism, regularly found in percomorph marine fishes, as reproductive style have been and are still subject of debate (Atz 1964, Smith 1967, 1975, Ghiselin 1969, Reinboth 1970, Policansky 1982). One clear advantage should be to maximize lifetime reproductive potential (Williams 1966) and hence individual fitness (*sensu* Stearns 1976). However, courtship, spawning, and sex change can be quite varied with mating systems in wrasses including haremic mating groups, promiscuity, lek-like behavior leading to group spawning, and facultative monogamy (pair spawning) (Donaldson, 1995). A change in sex is often associated with a change in color pattern. Broadcast spawning is a general rule in the Labridae, with most species being characterized by planktonic eggs and larvae and therefore a lack of any kind of brood care behavior, a pattern typical for the majority of marine fish species. In contrast, brood care is well developed in the comparatively small wrasse tribe Labrini (Hanel *et al.* 2002). Labrine wrasses show a variety of different brood care strategies, representing evolutionary succession from simple formation of spawning cavities up to the construction of complex nests associated with extensive egg care performed by territorial males and supported by one to several "helpers". Nevertheless, the effect of different brood care strategies on population size and structure as well as on phylogeography has, to our knowledge, not yet been tested.

CONCLUSION

Over the past two decades, fishes have emerged as excellent model groups for the study of phylogeography, speciation and adaptive radiation. This is not least due to their well-defined habitats, the existence of strong migration barriers bordering their living space, their restricted possibilities for migration and dispersal, and the availability of genetic tools. Different groups of fishes vary with respect to phylogeography and population structure: An extensive literature review revealed substantial differences in the geographic distances over which gene flow was detected in various groups of fishes that inhabit diverse environments. Marine fish typically show low to non-existing gene flow over hundreds to thousands of kilometers, while populations of lacustrine fishes, such as the cichlid fishes in the East African Great Lakes, are typically highly structured.

Box 1: The adaptive radiations of cichlid fishes

The perciform family of the Cichlidae represents a group of tropical and subtropical freshwater fish that show an Gondwanian distribution with ancestral and relatively species-poor lineages in India, Sri Lanka and Madagscar and two highly diverse clades in South- and Central America and in Africa, respectively (Salzburger & Meyer 2004). The most impressive cichlid adaptive radiations have occurred in the East African Great Lakes where at least 1500 species have evolved in the last few millions to several thousands of years only (Kocher 2004; Seehausen 2006; Salzburger 2009). Various hypotheses exist with respect to the evolutionary success of this group, and it seems likely that a unique combination of intrinsic (biotic) and extrinsic (abiotic) factors have triggered their adaptive radiations (Salzburger 2009). It has long been suggested that the particular architecture of the cichlid's jaw apparatus – with a second set of jaws in the pharynx – has acted as evolutionary key innovation in the adaptive radiations cichlids (Liem 1973). The most species-rich group of cichlids, the haplochromines from East Africa, are characterized by their particular kind of maternal mouthbrooding and egg-dummies on the male anal fins, which mimic real eggs and aid to bring the females mouth close to the male's genital opening. Both maternal mouthbrooding and egg-dummies might have acted as key-innovations, too (Salzburger *et al.* 2005; Salzburger 2009). It appears that both, ecologically relevant and, hence, naturally selected traits (*e.g.* moth morphology, body shape) and sexually selected traits (*e.g.* coloration) are important during cichlid speciation (Salzburger 2009).

Possible extrinsic factors are repeatedly occurring fluctuations of the lake level and the habitat diversity found in the East African lakes (Sturmbauer 1998; Kornfield & Smith 2000; Sturmbauer *et al.* 2001). Habitat discontinuities, together with often philopatric and stenotopic behavior of many of the cichlid species, may be partly responsible for their explosive speciation in lakes Victoria, Malawi and Tanganyika (van Oppen *et al.* 1997; Rico & Turner 2002; Rico *et al.* 2003; Pereyra *et al.* 2004; Duftner *et al.* 2006; Sefc *et al.* 2007).

Number of species (estimated): 3000-5000
Distribution range: Gondwanian (India, Sri Lanka, Madagascar, Africa, South- and Central America)
Habitat: freshwater (lakes and rivers)
Key-innovations (suggested): pharyngeal jaw apparatus, egg-dummies

Box 2: The adaptive radiation of notothenioids

Fishes of the perciform suborder Notothenioidei have successfully colonized the Antarctic waters and radiated under these harsh conditions. Today, the notothenioids dominate the Antarctic continental shelf and upper slope in terms of species number (47%) and biomass (90-95%) (Eastman & Clarke, 1998). Estimates for the onset of the notothenioid radiation range between 24 (Near 2004) and 7-15 MYA (Bargelloni *et al.* 1994; Cheng *et al.* 2003). Today, eight families and at least 130 notothenioid species are known. The three basal families, Bovichtidae, Pseudaphritidae and Eleginopidae comprise 13 species, 12 of which are non-Antarctic and occur in the coastal waters of New Zealand, Australia and around the tip of South America. The five remaining families Nototheniidae, Harpagiferidae, Artedidraconidae, Bathydraconidae and Channichthyidae consist of 116 mainly Antarctic species (Eastman 2005). Typically, only the latter five families (the 'Antarctic clade') are referred to when speaking of the notothenioid radiation.

The remarkable diversification of the Notothenioidei has been accompanied by several innovations in physiology. The most general feature found in all notothenioids, but not in higher-level relatives, is a lack of swim bladders. For this reason, most notothenioids are heavier than seawater and dwell on or near the seafloor. However, several notothenioid lineages have independently colonized the water column in a trend termed pelagization (Klingenberg & Ekau 1996). The expression of heat-shock proteins (HSPs) as a response to elevated temperatures, a feature that is regarded as a universal characteristic of almost all organisms, has been found absent in the highly cold-adapted members of the Antarctic clade (Hofmann *et al.* 2000; Clark *et al.* 2008). Recently, it has been shown that members of the Antarctic clade lack the mitochondrial *ND6* gene (coding for the NADH-Dehydrogenase subunit 6) (Papetti *et al.* 2007a). All members of the most derived notothenioid family, the Channichthyidae, have lost the ability to synthesize hemoglobin (Ruud 1954; Eastman 1993), and thus represent the only vertebrates without oxygen-bearing blood pigments. While the absence of hemoglobin is due to the deletion of the β-globin subunit gene in a single deletion event (di Prisco *et al.* 2002), truncated and inactive remnants of the α-globin gene are retained in channichthyid genomes (Cocca *et al.* 1995; Near *et al.* 2006). Since the oxygen-carrying capacity of the hemoglobinless phenotype is reduced by a factor of ten, the Channichthyidae evolved compensational features such as a blood volume two to four times that of comparable teleosts, a large stroke volume and cardiac output, and relatively large diameters of arteries and capillaries (Eastman 1993).

The most remarkable innovation of notothenioids are special blood-borne antifreeze glycoproteins (AFGPs), that are present in all notothenioids of the Antarctic clade, and enable them to cope with the subzero temperatures of Antarctic waters (Cheng *et al.* 2003). There is evidence that the AFGPs evolved only once in notothenioids from a trypsinogen ancestor gene, and that this happened before the diversification of the Antarctic clade (Chen *et al.* 1997; Cheng *et al.* 2003). It is thus tempting to attribute the notothenioid radiation to the evolution of AFGPs as a key adaptation with respect to the cooling environment. It may have enabled the notothenioids to survive the temperature drop in Antarctic waters from around 20°C to the current freezing conditions (Clarke & Johnston 1996), and to radiate while most other teleosts could not adapt to the decreasing temperatures.

Number of species: ca. 130
Distribution range: Antratctic waters, South Pacific
Habitat: polar marine
Key-innovations (suggested): antifreeze glycoproteins

Box 3: The (adaptive) radiation of labrids

The perciform family Labridae is a diverse group of about 600 mostly reef-dwelling species in 82 genera that exhibit an exceptional diversity in body size, shape, coloration, feeding habits, reproductive behaviors, and life histories (Westneat 1999, Parenti & Randall 2000, Wainwright *et al.* 2004, Westneat & Alfaro 2005). Together with the parrotfishes (Scaridae) as well as the cales and weed-whitings (Odacidae), which were all shown to be deeply nested within the Labridae (Bellwood 1994, Westneat and Alfaro 2005), wrasses comprise the worldwide second largest family of marine fish.

As with many percoid families the fossil record of the Labridae extends back to the Eocene (Lower Tertiary, approx. 54 MYA) (Berg 1958; Patterson, 1993) with †*Phyllopharyngodon longipinnis* Bellwood 1990 being described from a specimen recovered from the Pesciara ("Fish Bowl") in Monte Bolca, Italy (Bellwood 1990). Being dated to topmost Ypresian or lowermost Lutetian (Benton *et al.* 1993), this results in an estimated age of about 48 to 50 MY (Luterbacher *et al.* 2004). Based on the presence of a single predorsal, a well-developed pharyngeal jaw, and the phyllodont form of the teeth found on the pharyngeal jaw, Bellwood (1990) placed the specimen with confidence among the basal wrasse clade Hypsigenyini. However, based on plate tectonics, dating of reef lineages with molecular clocks and patterns of fish otolith preservation, the overall age of the family is estimated to be anywhere between 50 and 90 MY (Bellwood & Wainwright 2002, Westneat & Alfaro 2005).

From an oceanographic point of view, this time period near the end of the Mesozoic and beginning of the Cenozoic was characterized by the continuation of the Gondwana break-up to form present-day shaped continents as well as the central role of the circum-tropical Tethys Sea connecting the Indian with the Atlantic Ocean.

Diversification of the Labridae has often been referred to as a consequence of the evolution of functional novelties in the feeding apparatus that have allowed them to occupy nearly every feeding guild in reef environments (Westneat & Alfaro 2005). Feeding habits in the group are as diverse as in cichlids, including specialized predation on gastropods, bivalves, crustaceans, fishes, coral mucous, zooplankton, ectoparasites, detritus and algae (Randall 1967, Westneat 1997). However, recent investigations point out that territorial behavior and strong sexual dichromatism, as expressed by many wrasse species, may effectively drive sexual selection and are therefore major factors for labrid diversification (Kazancioglu *et al.* 2009).

Number of species (estimated): 600
Distribution range: global
Habitat: tropical to temperate marine
Key-innovations (suggested): pharyngeal jaw apparatus

Three groups of the highly diverse perciform fishes that underwent adaptive radiations are the cichlids, the notothenioids and the labrids. They radiated in large freshwater lakes, the polar waters of Antarctica, and tropical to temperate marine environments, respectively. Speciation and diversification in all three groups has been connected to external factors such as habitat instability, and paleo-geological and paleo-climatological processes, and all three radiations have been associated with evolutionary key-innovations. Still, they differ in overall within-species phylogeography, in population structure and patterns and levels of gene flow. The marine representatives are also generally less specialized than the cichlids. Whether this is due to differences in life-history traits, such as breeding behavior, would need to be investigated.

ACKNOWLEDGMENTS

We would like to acknowledge our respective grant sponsors, the VolkswagenStiftung to MM, the German Science Foundation (DFG) to RH, and the Swiss National Science Foundation (SNF) and the European Research Council (ERC) to WS.

REFERENCES

*Abila R, Barluenga M, Engelken J, Meyer A, Salzburger W, (2004) Population-structure and genetic diversity in a haplochromine fish cichlid of a satellite lake of Lake Victoria. *Molecular Ecology* 13 (9), 2589-2602.

*Appleyard SA, Williams R, Ward RD, (2004) Population genetic structure of Patagonian toothfish in the West Indian sector of the Southern Ocean. *CCAMLR Science* 11, 12-32.

*Arnegard ME, Markert JA, Danley PD, Stauffer JR, Ambali AJ, Kocher, TD, (1999) Population structure and colour variation of the cichlid fish *Labeotropheus fuelleborni* Ahl along a recently formed archipelago of rocky habitat patches in southern Lake Malawi. *Proc R Soc Lond B Biol Sci* 266, 119-130.

Atz JW, (1964) Intersexuality in fishes. In: *Intersexuality in vertebrates including man* (eds. Marshall AJ, Armstrong CN) pp. 145-232. Academic Press, NY.

*Aurelle D, Guillemaud T, Afonso P, Morato T, Wirtz P, Santos RS, Cancela ML, (2003) Genetic study of *Coris julis* (Osteichtyes, Perciformes, Labridae) evolutionary history and dispersal abilities. *Comptes Rendus Biologies* 326, 771-785.

Avise JC, (1998) The history and purview of phylogeography: a personal reflection. *Molecular Ecology* 7, 371-379.

Avise JC, (2000) *Phylogeography: the history and formation of species.* Harvard University Press, Cambridge, MA.

Avise JC, (2009) Phylogeography: retrospect and prospect. *Journal of Biogeography* 36, 3-15.

Avise JC, Arnold J, Ball RM, Bermingham E, Lamb T, Neigel JE, Reeb CA, Saunders NC (1987) Intraspecific phylogeography: the mitochondrial DNA bridge between population genetics and systematics. *Annual Review of Ecology and Systematics* 18, 489-522.

*Baerwald MR, Feyrer F, May B, (2008) Distribution of genetically differentiated splittail populations during the nonspawning season. *Transactions of the American Fisheries Society* 137 (5), 1335-1345.

Bargelloni L, Ritchie PA, Patarnello T, Battaglia B, Lambert DM, Meyer A, (1994) Molecular evolution at subzero temperatures: mitochondrial and nuclear phylogenies of fishes from Antarctica (suborder Notothenioidei), and the evolution of antifreeze glycopeptides. *Molecular Biology and Evolution* 11 (6), 854-863.

Barlow GW, (2000) *The Cichlid Fishes. Nature's Grand Experiment in Evolution.* Perseus Publishing, Cambridge, MA.

Barluenga M, Meyer A, (2004) The Midas cichlid species complex: incipient sympatric speciation in Nicaraguan cichlid fishes? *Mol Ecol* 13, 2061-2076.

Barluenga M, Stolting KN, Salzburger W, Muschick M, Meyer A, (2006) Sympatric speciation in Nicaraguan crater lake cichlid fish. *Nature* 439, 719-723.

Barnes DKA, Conlan KE, (2007) Disturbance, colonization and development of Antarctic benthic communities. *Philosophical Transactions of the Royal Society of London B: Biological Sciences* 362 (1477), 11-38.

*Barroso RM, Hilsdorf AWS, Modeira HLM, Cabello PH, Traub-Cseko YM, (2005) Genetic diversity of wild and cultured populations of *Brycon opalinus* (Cuvier, 1819) (Characiforme, Characidae, Bryconiae) using microsatellites. *Aquaculture* 247, 51-65.

*Barson NJ, Cable J, van Oosterhout C, (2009) Population genetic analysis of microsatellite variation of guppies (*Poecilia reticulata*) in Trinidad and Tobago: evidence for a dynamic source-sink metapopulation structure, founder events and population bottlenecks. *Journal of Evolutionary Biology* 22 (3), 485-497.

*Batista JS, Alves-Gomes JA, (2006) Phylogeography of *Brachyplatystoma rousseauxii* (Siluriformes - Pimelodidae) in the Amazon Basin offers preliminary evidence for the first case of "homing" for an Amazonian migratory catfish. *Genetics and Molecular Research* 5 (4), 723-740.

*Bay LK, Caley MJM, Crozier RH, (2008) Meta-population structure in a coral reef fish demonstrated by genetic data on patterns of migration, extinction and re-colonisation. *BMC Evolutionary Biology* 8 (1), 248.

Bellwood DR, (1990) A new fossil fish *Phyllopharyngodon longipinnis* gen. et sp. nov. (family Labridae) from the Eocene, Monte Bolca, Italy. *Studi e Ricerche sui Giacimenti Terziari di Bolca* 6, 149-160.

Bellwood DR, (1994) A phylogenetic study of the parrotfishes family Scaridae (Pisces:Labroidei), with a revision of genera. *Records of the Australian Museum Supplement* 20, 1-86.

Bellwood DR, Wainwright PC (2002) The history and biogeography of fishes on coral reefs. In: *Coral reef fishes: dynamics and diversity in a complex ecosystem* (ed. Sale PF), pp. 5-32. Academic Press San Diego, CA.

Benjamini Y, Hochberg Y, (1995) Controlling the false discovery rate: a practical and powerful approach to multiple testing. *Journal of the Royal Society B: Methodological* 57 (1), 289-300.

Benton MJ, (1993) *The Fossil record 2*. Chapman & Hall, London, UK.

Berg LS, (1958) *System der rezenten und fossilen Fischartigen und Fische*. VEB Verlag der Wissenschaften, Berlin.

Bernatchez L, Chouinard A, Guoqing L, (1999) Integrating molecular genetics and ecology in studies of adaptive radiation: whitefish, *Coregonus* sp., as a case study. *Biological Journal of the Linnean Society* 68, 173-194.

Bernatchez L, Wilson CC, (1998) Comparative phylogeography of Nearctic and Palearctic fishes. *Molecular Ecology* 7, 431-452.

Bouton N, Witte F, van Alphen JJ, Seehausen O, (1999) Local adaptations in populations of rock-dewlling haplochromines (Pisces: Cichlidae) from southern Lake Victoria. *Proc R Soc Lond B Biol Sci* 266, 366-360.

Brenner M, Buck B, Cordes S, Dietrich L, Jacob U, Mintenbeck K, Schröder A, Brey T, Knust R, Arntz WE, (2001) The role of iceberg scours in niche separation within the Antarctic fish genus *Trematomus*. *Polar Biology* 24 (7), 502-507.

*Caldera EJ, Bolnick DI (2008) Effects of colonization history and landscape structure on genetic variation within and among threespine stickleback (*Gasterosteus aculeatus*) populations in a single watershed. *Evolutionary Ecology Research* 10, 575-598.

Carreras-Carbonell J, Macpherson E, Pascual M (2005) Rapid radiation and cryptic speciation in mediterranean triplefin blennies (Pisces: Tripterygiidae) combining multiple genes. *Molecular Phylogenetics and Evolution* 37 (3), 751-761.

*Carvalho-Costa LF, Hatanka T, Galetti Jr. PM (2008) Evidence of lack of population substructuring in the Brazilian freshwater fish *Prochilodus costatus*. *Genetics and Molecular Biology* 31 (1), 377-380.

*Chabot CL, Allen LG (2009) Global population structure of the tope (*Galeorhinus galeus*) inferred by mitochondrial control region sequence data. *Molecular Ecology* 18, 545-552.

*Chauhan T, Lal KK, Mohindra V, Singh R, Punia P, Gopalakrishnan A, Sharma PC, Lakra W (2007) Evaluating genetic differentiation in wild populations of the Indian major carp, *Cirrhinus mrigala* (Hamilton-Buchanan, 1882): Evidence from allozyme and microsatellite markers. *Aquaculture* 269, 135-149.

Chen L, DeVries AL, Cheng, CHC (1997) Evolution of antifreeze glycoprotein gene from a trypsinogen gene in Antarctic notothenioid fish. *PNAS* 94 (8), 3811-3816.

*Chen S, Liu T, Li Z, Gao T (2008) Genetic population structuring and demographic history of red spotted grouper (*Epinephelus akaara*) in South and East China Sea. *African Journal of Biotechnology* 7 (20), 3554-3562.

Cheng CHC, Chen L, Near TJ, Jin Y (2003) Functional antifreeze glycoprotein genes in temperate-water New Zealand nototheniid fish infer an Antarctic evolutionary origin. *Molecular Biology and Evolution* 20 (11), 1897-1908.

*Chow S, Suzuki N, Brodeur RD, Ueno Y (2009) Little population structuring and recent evolution of the Pacific saury (*Cololabis saira*) as indicated by mitochondrial and nuclear DNA sequence data. *Journal of Experimental Marine Biology and Ecology* 369, 17-21.

Clark MS, Fraser KPP, Burns G, Peck LS (2008) The HSP70 heat shock response in the Antarctic fish *Harpagifer antarcticus*. *Polar Biology* 31 (2), 171-180.

Clarke A, Johnston IA (1996) Evolution and adaptive radiation of antarctic fishes. *Trends in Ecology and Evolution* 11 (5), 212-218.

Cocca E, Ratnayake-Lecamwasam M, Parker SK, Camardella L, Ciaramella M, di Prisco G, Detrich III HW (1995) Genomic remnants of alpha-globin genes in the hemoglobinless antarctic icefishes. *PNAS* 92 (6), 1817-1821.

Cohen AS, Lezzar KE, Tiercelin JJ, Soreghan M (1997) New paleogeographic and lake-level reconstructions of Lake Tanganyika: implications for tectonic, climatic and biological evolution in a rift lake. *Basin Research* 7, 107-132.

Coyne JA, Orr HA (2004) *Speciation* Sinauer Associates, Sunderland, Massachusetts.

*Craig MT, Eble JA, Bowen BW, Robertson DR (2007) High genetic connectivity across the Indian and Pacific Oceans in the reef fish *Myripristis berndti* (Holocentridae). *Marine Ecology Progress Series* 334, 245-254.

Crandall KA, Bininda-Emonds ORP, Mace GM, Wayne RK (2000) Considering evolutionary processes in conservation biology. *Trends in Ecology and Evolution* 15 (7), 290-295.

*Curley BG, Gillings MR (2009) Population connectivity in the temperate damselfish *Parma microlepis*: analyses of genetic structure across multiple spatial scales. *Marine Biology* 156 (3), 381-393.

*Danancher D, Izquierdo JI, Garcia-Vazquez E (2008) Microsatellite analysis of relatedness structure in young of the year of the endangered *Zingel asper* (Percidae) and implications for conservation. *Freshwater Biology* 53 (3), 546-557.

Dawson MN, Waples RS, Bernardi (2006) Phylogeography. In: *The Ecology of Marine Fishes* (eds. Allan LG, Pondella DJ, Horn MH), pp. 26-54. University of California Press, CA.

Debes PV, Zachos FE, Hanel R (2008) Mitochondrial phylogeography of the European sprat (*Sprattus sprattus* L., Clupeidae) reveals isolated climatically vulnerable populations in the Mediterranean Sea and range expansion in the northeast Atlantic. *Molecular Ecology* 17, 3873-3888.

de Graaf M, Dejen E, Osse JWM, Sibbing FA (2008) Adaptive radiation of Lake Tana's (Ethiopia) *Labeobarbus* species flock (Pisces, Cyprinidae). *Marine and Freshwater Research* 59, 391-407.

Dieckmann U, Doebeli M (1999) On the origin of species by sympatric speciation. *Nature* 400, 354-357.

*Dillane E, Cross MC, McGinnity P, Coughlan JP, Galvin PT, Wilkins NP, Cross TF (2007) Spatial and temporal patterns in microsatellite DNA variation of wild Atlantic salmon, *Salmo salar*, in Irish rivers. *Fisheries Management and Ecology* 14, 209-219.

*Dillane E, McGinnity P, Coughlan JP, Cross MC, de Eyto E, Kenchington E, Prodöhl P, Cross TF (2008) Demographics and landscape features determine intrariver population structure in Atlantic salmon (*Salmo salar* L.): the case of the River Moy in Ireland. *Molecular Ecology* 17 (22), 4786-4800.

Dimitrov D, Arnedo MA, Ribera C (2008) Colonization and diversification of the spider genus *Pholcus* Walckenaer, 1805 (Araneae, Pholcidae) in the Macaronesian archipelagos: evidence for long-term occupancy yet rapid recent speciation. *Molecular Phylogenetics and Evolution* 48, 596-614.

di Prisco G, Cocca E, Parker SK, Detrich III HW (2002) Tracking the evolutionary loss of hemoglobin expression by the white-blooded Antarctic icefishes. *Gene* 295 (2), 185-191.

Donaldson TJ (1995). Courtship and spawning of nine species of wrasses (Labridae) from the western Pacific. *Jap J Ichthyol* 42, 311-319.

*Drew J, Allen GR, Kaufmann L, Barber PH (2008) Endemism and regional color and genetic differences in five putatively cosmopolitan reef fishes. *Conservation Biology* 22 (4), 965-975.

*Dudgeon CL, Broderick D, Ovenden JR (2009) IUCN classification zones concord with, but underestimate, the population genetic structure of the zebra shark *Stegostoma fasciatum* in the Indo-West Pacific. *Molecular Ecology* 18 (2), 248-261.

*Duftner N, Sefc KM, Koblmuller S, Nevado B, Verheyen E, Phiri H, Sturmbauer C (2006) Distinct population structure in a phenotypically homogeneous rock-dwelling cichlid fish from Lake Tanganyika. *Mol Ecol* 15, 2381-2395.

Eastman JT (1993) *Antarctic fish biology: evolution in a unique environment*. Academic Press, San Diego, CA.

Eastman JT (2005) The nature of the diversity of Antarctic fishes. *Polar Biology* 28, 93-107.

Eastman JT, Clarke A (1998) A comparison of adaptive radiations of Antarctic fish with those of non-Antarctic fish. In: *Fishes of Antarctica. A biological overview* (eds. di Prisco G, Pisano E, Clarke A), pp. 3-26. Springer, Milan, Italy.

*Eble JA, Toonen RJ, Bowen BW (2009) Endemism and dispersal: comparative phylogeography of three surgeonfishes across the Hawaiian Archipelago. *Marine Biology* 156 (4), 689-698.

*Elmer KR, van Houdt JKJ, Meyer A, Volckaert FAM (2008) Population genetic structure of North American burbot (*Lota lota maculosa*) across the Nearctic and at its contact zone with Eurasian burbot (*Lota lota lota*). *Canadian Journal of Fisheries and Aquatic Sciences* 65 (11), 2412-2426.

Evans CW, Cziko PA, Cheng CHC, DeVries AL (2005) Spawning behaviour and early development in the naked dragonfish *Gymnodraco acuticeps*. *Antarctic Science* 17 (3), 319-327.

Feulner PG, Kirschbaum F, Mamonekene V, Ketmaier V, Tiedemann R (2007) Adaptive radiation in African weakly electric fish (Teleostei: Mormyridae: Campylomormyrus): a combined molecular and morphological approach. *J Evol Biol* 20, 403-414.

Floeter SR, Rocha LA, Robertson DR, *et al.* (2008) Atlantic reef fish biogeography and evolution. *Journal of Biogeography* 35, 22-47.

*Fontaine PM, Dodson JJ, Bernatchez L, Slettan A (1997) A genetic test of metapopulation structure in Atlantic salmon (*Salmo salar*) using microsatellites. *Canadian Journal of Fisheries and Aquatic Sciences* 54 2434-2442.

*Francisco SM, Cabral H, Vieira MN, Almada VC (2006) Contrasts in genetic structure and historical demography of marine and riverine populations of *Atherina* at similar geographical scales. *Estuarine, Coastal and Shelf Science* 69, 655-661.

*Froukh T, Kochzius M (2007) Genetic population structure of the endemic fourline wrasse (*Larabicus quadrilineatus*) suggests limited larval dispersal distances in the Red Sea. *Molecular Ecology* 16, 1359-1367.

*Galarza JA, Carbonell-Carreras J, Macpherson E, Pascual M, Roques S, Turner G, Rico C (2009) The influence of oceanographic fronts and early-life-history traits on connectivity among littoral fish species. *PNAS* 106 (5), 1473-1478.

Garant D, Forde SE, Hendry AP (2007) The multifarious effects of dispersal and gene flow on contemporary adaptation. *Functional Ecology* 21 (3), 434-443.

Gavrilets S (2004) *Fitness landscapes and the origin of species.* Princeton University Press, Princeton, New Jersey.

Gavrilets S, Vose A (2005) Dynamic patterns of adaptive radiation. *Proc Natl Acad Sci U S A* 102, 18040-18045.

Gavrilets S, Vose A, Barluenga M, Salzburger W, Meyer A (2007) Case studies and mathematical models of ecological speciation. 1. Cichlids in a crater lake. *Mol Ecol* 16, 2893-2909.

Ghiselin MT (1969) The evolution of hermaphroditism among animals. *Q Rev Biol* 44, 189-208.

Goodwin NB, Balshine-Earn S, Reynolds JD (1998) Evolutionary transitions in parental care in cichlid fish. *Proc R Soc Lond B Biol Sci* 265, 2265-2272.

*Goswami M, Thangaraj K, Chaudhary BK, Bjaskar, LVSK, Gopalakrishnan A, Joshi MB, Singh L, Lakra WS (2009) Genetic heterogeneity in the Indian stocks of seahorse

(*Hippocampus kuda* and *Hippocampus trimaculatus*) inferred from mtDNA cytochrome b gene. *Hydrobiologia* 621, 213-221.

Grant PR, Grant BR (2002) Unpredictable evolution in a 30-year study of Darwin's finches. *Science* 296, 707-711.

Grant PR, Grant BR (2006) Evolution of character displacement in Darwin's finches. *Science* 313, 224-226.

*Grunwald C, Stabile J, Waldman JR, Gross R, Wirgin I (2002) Population genetics of shortnose sturgeon *Acipenser brevirostrum* based on mitochondrial DNA control region sequences. *Molecular Ecology* 11, 1885-1898.

*Grunwald C, Maceda L, Waldman JR, Stabile J, Wirgin I (2008) Conservation of Atlantic sturgeon *Acipenser oxyrinchus oxyrinchus*: delineation of stock structure and distinct population segments. *Conservation Genetics* 9, 1111-1124.

*Guy TJ, Gresswell RE, Banks MA (2008) Landscape-scale evaluation of genetic structure among barrier-isolated populations of coastal cutthroat trout, *Oncorhynchus clarkii clarkii*. *Canadian Journal of Fisheries and Aquatic Sciences* 65, 1749-1762.

Hanel R, Westneat MW, Sturmbauer C (2002)Phylogenetic relationships, evolution of broodcare behavior, and geographic speciation in the Wrasse tribe Labrini. *Journal of Molecular Evolution* 55, 776-789.

*Hatanaka T, Henrique-Silva F, Galetti Jr. PM (2006) Population Substructuring in a Migratory Freshwater Fish Prochilodus argenteus (Characiformes, Prochilodontidae) from the São Francisco River. *Genetica* 126, 153-159.

*Hepburn RI, Sale PF, Dixon B, Heath DD (2009) Genetic structure of juvenile cohorts of bicolor damselfish (*Stegastes partitus*) along the Mesoamerican barrier reef: chaos through time. *Coral Reefs* 28 (1), 277-288.

Herder F, Nolte AW, Pfaender J, Schwarzer J, Hadiaty RK, Schliewen UK (2006) Adaptive radiation and hybridization in Wallace's Dreamponds: evidence from sailfin silversides in the Malili Lakes of Sulawesi. *Proc Biol Sci* 273, 2209-2217.

Hey J, Nielsen R (2007) Integration within the Felsenstein equation for improved Markov chain Monte Carlo methods in population genetics. *PNAS* 104 (8), 2785-2790.

*Hickey AJR, Lavery SD, Hannan DA, Baker CS, Clements KD (2009) New Zealand triplefin fishes (family Tripterygiidae): contrasting population structure and mtDNA diversity within a marine species flock. *Molecular Ecology* 18, 680-696.

Higashi M, Takimoto G, Yamamura N (1999) Sympatric speciation by sexual selection. *Nature* 402, 523-526.

Hofmann GE, Buckley BA, Airaksinen S, Keen JE, Somero GN (2000) Heat-shock protein expression is absent in the antarctic fish Trematomus bernacchii (family Nototheniidae). *Journal of Experimental Biology* 203 (15), 2331-2339.

*Horne JB, van Herwerden L, Choat JH, Robertson DR (2008) High population connectivity across the Indo-Pacific: Congruent lack of phylogeographic structure in three reef fish congeners. *Molecular Phylogenetics and Evolution* 49 (2), 629-638.

*Hrbek T, Farias IP, Crossa M, Sampaio I, Porto JIR, Meyer A (2005) Population genetic analysis of *Arapaima gigas*, one of the largest freshwater fishes of the Amazon basin: implications for its conservation. *Animal Conservation* 8, 297-308.

Hsü KJ, Montadert L, Bernoulli D, Cita MB, Erickson A, Garrison RE, Kidd RB, Mèlierés F, Müller C, Wright R (1977) History of the Mediterranean salinity crisis. *Nature* 267, 399-403.

Hsü KJ, Ryan WBF, Cita MB (1973) Late Miocene desiccation of the Mediterranean. *Nature* 242, 240-244.

*Hubert N, Duponchelle F, Nuñez J, Rivera R, Bonhomme F, Renno JF (2007) Isolation by distance and Pleistocene expansion of the lowland populations of the white piranha *Serrasalmus rhombeus*. *Molecular Ecology* 16, 2488-2503.

Hulsey (2006) Function of a key morphological innovation: fusion of the cichlid pharyngeal jaw. *Proc Biol Sci* 263, 669-675.

Janko K, Lecointre G, DeVries AL, Couloux A, Cruaud C, Marshall C (2007) Did glacial advances during the Pleistocene influence differently the demographic histories of benthic and pelagic Antarctic shelf fishes? - Inferences from intraspecific mitochondrial and nuclear DNA sequence diversity. *BMC Evolutionary Biology* 7, 220.

Johnson TC, Scholz CA, Talbot MR, Kelts K, Ricketts RD, Ngobi G, Beuning K, Ssemmanda II, McGill JW (1996) Late Pleistocene Desiccation of Lake Victoria and Rapid Evolution of Cichlid Fishes. *Science* 273, 1091-1093.

*Jones CD, Anderson ME, Balushkin AV, Duhamel G, Eakin RR, Eastman JT, Kuhn KL, Lecointre G, Near TJ, North AW, Stein DL, Vacchi M, Detrich III HW (2008) Diversity, relative abundance, new locality records and population structure of Antarctic demersal fishes from the northern Scotia Arc islands and Bouvetøya. *Polar Biology* 31, 1481-1497.

Juan C, Ibrahim KM, Oromí P, Hewitt GM (1998) The phylogeography of the darkling beetle, *Hegeter politus*, in the eastern Canary Islands. *Proceedings of the Royal Society of London B: Biological Sciences* 265 (1391), 135-140.

Kazancioglu E, Near TJ, Hanel R, Wainwright PC (2009) Influence of feeding functual morphology and sexual selection on diversification rate of parrotfishes (Scaridae). Submitted to *Proceedings of the Royal Society B*.

Kellermann AK (1991) Egg and larval drift of the Antarctic fish *Notothenia coriiceps*. *Cybium* 15 (3), 199-210.

*Kitanishi S, Yamamoto T, Higashi S (2009) Microsatellite variation reveals fine-scale genetic structure of masu salmon, *Oncorhynchus masou*, within the Atsuta River. *Ecology of Freshwater Fish* 18, 65-71.

Klingenberg CP, Ekau W (1996) A combined morphometric and phylogenetic analysis of an ecomorphological trend: pelagization in Antarctic fishes (Perciformes: Nototheniidae). *Biological Journal of the Linnean Society* 59, 143-177.

Kocher TD (2004) Adaptive evolution and explosive speciation: the cichlid fish model. *Nature Reviews Genetics* 5, 288-298.

Kock KH (2005) Antarctic icefishes (Channichthyidae): a unique family of fishes. A review, part I. *Polar Biology* 28 (11), 862-895.

Kock KH, Kellermann AK (1991) Reproduction in Antarctic notothenioid fish. *Antarctic Science* 3 (2), 125-150.

Kock KH, Pshenichnov LK, DeVries AL (2006) Evidence for egg brooding and parental care in icefish and other notothenioids in the Southern Ocean. *Antarctic Science* 18 (2), 223-227.

Kondrashov AS, Kondrashov FA (1999) Interactions among quantitative traits in the course of sympatric speciation. *Nature* 400, 351-354.

Kornfield I, Carpenter KE (1984) Cyprinids of Lake Lanao, Philippines: Taxonomic validity, evolutionary rates and speciation scenarios. In: *Evolution of Fish Species Flocks* (eds. Echelle AA, Kornfield I), pp. 69-84. University of Maine at Orono Press, Orono, Maine.

Kornfield I, Smith PF (2000) African Cichlid Fishes: Model systems for evolutionary biology. *Annu. Rev. Ecol. Syst.* 31, 163-196.

*Kuhn KL, Gaffney PM (2006) Preliminary assessment of population structure in the mackerel icefish (*Champsocephalus gunnari*). *Polar Biology* 29, 927-935.

La Mesa M, Ashford J (2008) Age and early life history of juvenile scotia sea icefish, *Chaenocephalus aceratus*, from Elephant and the South Shetland Islands. *Polar Biology* 31 (2), 221-228.

Leis JM (2006) Are larvae of demersal fishes plankton or nekton? *Advances in Marine Biology* 51, 57-141.

Lessios HA (1998) The first stage of speciation as seen in organisms separated by the Isthmus of Panama. In: *Endless Forms: Species and Speciation* (eds. Howard DH, Berlocher SH), pp. 186-201. Oxord University Press, Oxford, UK.

Liem KF (1973) Evolutionary strategies and morphological innovations: cichlid pharyngeal jaws. *Systematic Zoology* 22, 425-441.

*Lin J, Quinn TP, Hilborn R, Hauser L (2008a) Fine-scale differentiation between sockeye salmon ecotypes and the effect of phenotype on straying. *Heredity* 101 (4), 341-350.

*Lin J, Zigeler E, Quinn TP, Hauser L (2008b) Contrasting patterns of morphological and neutral genetic divergence among geographically proximate populations of sockeye salmon *Oncorhynchus nerka* in Lake Aleknagik, Alaska. *Journal of Fish Biology* 73 (8), 1993-2004.

Loeb VJ, Kellermann AK, Koubbi P, North AW, White MG (1993) Antarctic larval fish assemblages: a review. *Bulletin of Marine Science* 53 (2), 416-449.

Lourie SA, Vincent ACJ (2004) A marine fish follows Wallace's Line: the phylogeography of the three-spot seahorse (*Hippocampus trimaculatus*, Syngnathidae, Teleostei) in Southeast Asia. *Journal of Biogeography* 31, 1975-1985.

Losos JB, Jackmann TR, Larson A, De Queiroz K, Rodrigues-Schettino L (1998) Contingency and determinism in replicated adaptive radiations of island lizards. *Science* 279, 2115-2118.

Luterbacher HP, Ali JR, Brinkhuis H, Gradstein FM, Hooker JJ, Monechi S, Ogg JG, Powell J, Röhl U, Sanfilippo A, Schmitz B (2004) The Paleogene period. In: *A geologic time scale* (ed. Gradstein F, Ogg J, Smith A), pp. 384-408. Cambridge University Press, Cambridge.

Mabuchi K, Miya M, Azuma Y, Nishida M (2007) Independent evolution of the specialized pharyngeal jaw apparatus in cichlid and labrid fishes. *BMC Evol Biol* 7, 10.

*Markert JA, Arnegard ME, Danley PD, Kocher TD (1999) Biogeography and population genetics of the Lake Malawi cichlid *Melanochromis auratus*: habitat transience, philopatry and speciation. *Molecular Ecology* 8, 1013-1026.

*Matschiner M, Hanel R, Salzburger W (2009) Gene flow by larval dispersal in the Antarctic notothenioid fish *Gobionotothen gibberifrons*. *Molecular Ecology*, in press.

Mayr E (1942) *Systematics and the Origin of Species* Columbia University Press, New York.

Mayr E (1963) *Animal Species and Evolution* Harvard University Press, Cambridge.

McCune AR (1997) How fast is speciation? Molecular, geological and phylogenetic evidence from adaptive radiations of fishes. In: *Molecular evolution and adaptive radiation* (eds. Givinish TJ, Sytsma KJ), pp. 585-610. Cambridge University Press, Cambridge, UK.

*Miller-Sims VC, Gerlach G, Kingsford MJ, Atema J (2008) Dispersal in the spiny damselfish, *Acanthochromis polyacanthus*, a coral reef fish species without a larval pelagic stage. *Molecular Ecology* 17 (23), 5036-5048.

Moritz C (1994) Defining 'Evolutionary Significant Units' for conservation. *Trends in Ecology and Evolution* 9 (10), 373-375.

Muss A, Robertson DR, Stepien CA, Wirtz P, Bowen BW (2001) Phylogeography of *Ophioblennius*: the role of ocean currents and geography in reef fish evolution. *Evolution* 55 (3), 561-572.

Mwanja WW, Armoudlian AS, Wandera SB, Kaufmann L, Wu L, Booton GC, Fuerst PA (2001) The bounty of minor lakes: the role of small satellite water bodies in evolution and conservation of fishes in the Lake Victoria Region, East Africa. *Hydrobiologia* 458, 55-62.

Near TJ (2004) Estimating divergence times of notothenioid fishes using a fossil-calibrated molecular clock. *Antarctic Science* 16, 37-44.

Near TJ, Cheng CHC (2008) Phylogenetics of notothenioid fishes (Teleostei: Acanthomorpha): inferences from mitochondrial and nuclear gene sequences. *Mol Phylogenet Evol* 47, 832-840.

Near TJ, Parker SK, Detrich III HW (2006) A genomic fossil reveals key steps in hemoglobin loss by the antarctic icefishes. *Molecular Biology and Evolution* 23 (11), 2008-2016.

*Neethling M, Matthee CA, Bowie RCK, von der Heyden S (2008) Evidence for panmixia despite barriers to gene flow in the southern African endemic, *Caffrogobius caffer* (Teleostei: Gobiidae). *BMC Evolutionary Biology* 8, 325.

Nelson JS (2006) *Fishes of the World.*

Nepokroeff M, Sytsma KJ, Wagner WL, Zimmer EA (2003) Reconstructing ancestral patterns of colonization and dispersal in the Hawaiian understory tree genus *Psychotria* (Rubiaceae): A comparison of parsimony and likelihood approaches. *Systematic Biology* 52 (6), 820-838.

*Osinov AG, Gordeeva NV (2008) Variability of the microsatellite DNA and genetic differentiation of the populations of residual form of Dolly varden trout *Salvelinus malma krascheninnikovi* of Sakhalin. *Journal of Ichthyology* 48 (9), 691-706.

Ostbye K, Bernatchez L, Naesje TF, Himberg KJ, Hindar K (2005) Evolutionary history of the European whitefish Coregonus lavaretus (L.) species complex as inferred from mtDNA phylogeography and gill-raker numbers. *Mol Ecol* 14, 4371-4387.

*Pálsson S, Källman T, Paulsen J, Árnason E (2009) An assessment of mitochondrial variation in Arctic gadoids. *Polar Biology* 32 (3), 471-479.

Palumbi SR (1994) Genetic divergence, reproductive isolation, and marine speciation. *Annual Review of Ecology and Systematics* 25, 547-572.

Papetti C, Liò P, Rüber L, Patarnello T, Zardoya R (2007a) Antarctic fish mitochondrial genomes lack ND6 gene. *Journal of Molecular Evolution* 65 (5), 519-528.

*Papetti C, Susana E, La Mesa M, Kock KH, Patarnello T, Zane L (2007b) Microsatellite analysis reveals genetic differentiation between year-classes in the icefish *Chaenocephalus aceratus* at South Shetlands and Elephant Island. *Polar Biology* 30 (12), 1605-1613.

Parenti LR (1984) Biogeography of the Andean killifish genus *Orestias* with comments on the species flock concept. In: *Evolution of Fish Species Flocks* (eds. Echelle AA, Kornfield I), pp. 85-92. University of Maine at Orono Press, Orono, Maine.

Parenti P, Randall JE (2000) An annotated checklist of the species of the labroid fish families Labridae and Scaridae. *Ichthyol. Bull. (J.L.B. Smith Inst.)* 68, 1–97.

*Patarnello T, Marcato S, Zane L, Varotto V, Bargelloni L (2003) Phylogeography of the Chionodraco genus (Perciformes, Channichthydae) in the Southern Ocean. *Molecular Phylogenetics and Evolution* 28, 420-429.

Patarnello T, Volckaert FJ, Castilho R (2007) Pillars of Hercules: is the Atlantic-Mediterranean transition a phylogeographical break? *Molecular Ecology* 16, 4426-4444.

Patterson C (1993) Vertebrates, Osteichthyes: Teleostei. In: *The fossil record 2* (ed. Benton MJ), pp. 621-657. Chapman & Hall, London, UK.

*Pereyra R, Taylor MI, Turner GF, Rico C (2004) Variation in habitat preference and population structure among three species of the Lake Malawi cichlid genus Protomelas. *Mol Ecol* 13, 2691-2697.

Policansky D (1982) Sex change in animals and plants. *Ann Rev Ecol Syst* 13, 471-495.

*Prodocimo V, Tschá MK, Pie MR, Oliveira-Neto JF, Ostrensky A, Boeger WA (2008) Lack of genetic differentiation in the fat snook *Centropomus parallelus* (Teleostei: Centropomidae) along the Brazilian coast. *Journal of Fish Biology* 73 (8), 2075-2082.

Puebla O, Bermingham E, Guichard F (2008) Population genetic analyses of Hypoplectrus coral reef fishes provide evidence that local processes are operating during the early stages of marine adaptive radiations. *Mol Ecol* 17, 1405-1415.

Puebla O, Bermingham E, Guichard F, Whiteman E (2007) Colour pattern as a single trait driving speciation in Hypoplectrus coral reef fishes? *Proc Biol Sci* 274, 1265-1271.

*Ramon ML, Nelson PA, Martini E, Walsh WJ, Bernardi G (2008) Phylogeography, historical demography, and the role of post-settlement ecology in two Hawaiian damselfish species. *Marine Biology* 153, 1207-1217.

Randall JE (1967) Food habits of reef fishes of the West Indies. *Stud Trop Oceanog (Miami)* 5, 655–847.

Reinboth R (1970) Intersexuality in fishes. *Mem Soc Endocr* 18, 515-543.

Rice WR (1989) Analysing tables of statistical tests. *Evolution* 43, 223-225.

Rico C, Bouteillon P, van Oppen MJ, Knight ME, Hewitt GM, Turner GF (2003) No evidence for parallel sympatric speciation in cichlid species of the genus *Pseudotropheus* from north-western Lake Malawi. *J Evol Biol* 16, 37-46.

*Rico C, Turner GF (2002) Extreme microallopatric divergence in a cichlid species from Lake Malawi. *Mol Ecol* 11, 1585-1590.

*Rivera MAJ, Kelley CD, Roderick GK (2004) Subtle population genetic structure in the Hawaiian grouper, *Epinephelus quernus* (Serranidae) as revealed by mitochondrial DNA analyses. *Biological Journal of the Linnean Society* 81, 449-468.

*Rocha LA, Bass AL, Robertson DR, Bowen BW (2002) Adult habitat preferences, larval dispersal, and the comparative phylogeography of three Atlantic surgeonfishes (Teleostei: Acanthuridae). *Molecular Ecology* 11, 243-252.

Rocha LA, Bowen BW (2008) Speciation in coral-reef fishes. *Journal of Fish Biology* 72, 1101-1121.

Rocha LA, Craig MT, Bowen BW (2007) Phylogeography and the conservation of coral reef fishes. *Coral Reefs* 26 (3), 501-512.

Rocha LA, Rocha CR, Robertson DR, Bowen BW (2008) Comparative phylogeography of Atlantic reef fishes indicates both origin and accumulation of diversity in the Caribbean. *BMC Evol Biol* 8, 157.

*Rogers AD, Morley S, Fitzcharles E, Jarvis K, Belchier M (2006) Genetic structure of Patagonian toothfish (*Dissostichus eleginoides*) populations on the Patagonian Shelf and Atlantic and western Indian Ocean Sectors of the Southern Ocean. *Marine Biology* 149, 915-924.

Rögl F (1999) Mediterranean and Paratethys. Facts and hypotheses of an Oligocene to Miocene palaeogeography (short overview). *Geologica Carpathica* 50 (4), 339-349.

Rossiter A (1995) The cichlid fish assemblages of Lake Tanganyika: ecology, behavior and evolution of its species flocks. *Advances in Ecological Research* 26, 157-252.

Roy D, Docker MF, Haffner GD, Heath DD (2007a) Body shape vs. colour associated initial divergence in the Telmatherina radiation in Lake Matano, Sulawesi, Indonesia. *J Evol Biol* 20, 1126-1137.

Roy D, Paterson G, Hamilton PB, Heath DD, Haffner GD (2007b) Resource-based adaptive divergence in the freshwater fish Telmatherina from Lake Matano, Indonesia. *Mol Ecol* 16, 35-48.

Rüber L, Van Tassell JL, Zardoya R (2003) Rapid speciation and ecological divergence in the American seven-spined gobies (Gobiidae, Gobiosomatini) inferred from a molecular phylogeny. *Evolution* 57, 1584-1598.

Rüber L, Zardoya R (2005) Rapid cladogenesis in marine fishes revisited. *Evolution Int J Org Evolution* 59, 1119-1127.

Ruud JT (1954) Vertebrates without erythrocytes and blood pigment. *Nature* 173 (4410), 848-850.

Ryder OA (1986) Species conservation and systematics: the dilemma of subspecies. *Trends in Ecology and Evolution.* 1, 9-10.

*Saito T, Washio S, Dairiki K, Shimojo M, Itoi S, Sugita H (2008) High gene flow in *Girella punctata* (Perciformes, Kyphosidae) among the Japanese Islands inferred from partial sequence of the control region in mitochondrial DNA. *Journal of Fish Biology* 73 (8), 1937-1945.

Salzburger W (2008) To be or not to be a hamlet pair in sympatry. *Mol Ecol* 17, 1397-1399.

Salzburger W (2009) The interaction of sexually and naturally selected traits in the adaptive radiations of cichlid fishes. *Mol Ecol* 18, 169-185.

Salzburger W, Brandstätter A, Gilles A, Parson W, Hempel M, Sturmbauer C, Meyer A (2003) Phylogeography of the vairone (*Leuciscus souffia*, Risso 1826) in Central Europe. *Molecular Ecology* 12 (9), 2371-2386.

Salzburger W, Mack T, Verheyen E, Meyer A (2005) Out of Tanganyika: Genesis, explosive speciation, key-innovations and phylogeography of the haplochromine cichlid fishes. *BMC Evolutionary Biology* 5, 17.

Salzburger W, Meyer A (2004) The species flocks of East African cichlid fishes: recent advances in molecular phylogenetics and population genetics. *Naturwissenschaften* 91, 277-290.

Sanchez S, Dettai A, Bonillo C, Ozouf-Costaz C, Detrich III HW, Lecointre G (2007) Molecular and morphological phylogenies of the Antarctic teleostean family Nototheniidae, with emphasis on the Trematominae. *Polar Biology* 30, 155-166.

*Santos MCF, Ruffino ML, Farias IP (2007) High levels of genetic variability and panmixia of the tambaqui *Colossoma macropomum* (Cuvier, 1816) in the main channel of the Amazon River. *Journal of Fish Biology* 71, 33-44.

Savolainen V, Anstett MC, Lexer C, *et al.* (2006) Sympatric speciation in palms on an oceanic island. *Nature* 441, 210-213.

Schliewen UK, Tautz D, Paabo S (1994) Sympatric speciation suggested by monophyly of crater lake cichlids. *Nature* 368, 629-632.

Schluter D (2000) *The Ecology of Adaptive Radiation* Oxford University Press, New York.

Schluter D, McPhail JD (1992) Ecological character displacement and speciation in sticklebacks. *American Naturalist* 140, 85-108.

*Schultz JK, Feldheim KA, Gruber SH, Ashley MV, McGovern TM, Bowen BW (2008) Global phylogeography and seascape genetics of the lemon sharks (genus *Negaprion*). *Molecular Ecology* 17 (24), 5336-5348.

Seehausen O (2002) Patterns in fish radiation are compatible with Pleistocene desiccation of Lake Victoria and 14,600 year history for its cichlid species flock. *Proc R Soc Lond B Biol Sci* 269, 491-470.

Seehausen O (2006) African cichlid fish: a model system in adaptive radiation research. *Proc Biol Sci* 273, 1987-1998.

*Sefc KM, Baric S, Salzburger W, Sturmbauer C (2007) Species-specific population structure in rock-specialized sympatric cichlid species in Lake Tanganyika, East Africa. *J Mol Evol* 64, 33-49.

Sequeira AS, Lanteri AA, Albelo LR, Bhattacharya S, Sijapati M (2008) Colonization history, ecological shifts and diversification in the evolution of endemic Galápagos weevils. *Molecular Ecology* 17 (4), 1089-1107.

Shaw KL (1996) Sequential Radiations and Patterns of Speciation in the Hawaiian Cricket Genus Laupala Inferred from DNA Sequences. *Evolution* 50 (1), 237-255.

*Shaw PW, Arkhipkin A, Al-Khairulla A (2004) Genetic structuring of Patagonian toothfish populations in the Southwest Atlantic Ocean: the effect of the Antarctic Polar Front and deep-water troughs as barriers to genetic exchange. *Molecular Ecology* 13, 3293-3303.

*Shaw PW, Turner GF, Idid MR, Robinson RL, Carvalho GR (2000) Genetic population structure indicates sympatric speciation of Lake Malawi pelagic cichlids. *Proc R Soc Lond B Biol Sci* 267, 2273-2280.

*Silva-Oliveira GC, do Rêgo PS, Schneider H, Sampaio I, Vallinoto M (2008) Genetic characterisation of populations of the critically endangered Goliath grouper (*Epinephelus itajara*, Serranidae) from the Northern Brazilian coast through analyses of mtDNA. *Genetics and Molecular Biology* 31 (4), 988-994.

Smith CL (1967) Contribution to a theory of hermaphroditism. *Journal of Theoretical Biology* 17, 76-90.

Smith CL (1975) The evolution of hermaphroditism in fishes. In: *Intersexuality in the Animal Kingdom* (ed. Reinboth R), pp. 295-310. Springer Verlag, New York.

*Smith PJ, Gaffney PM (2005) Low genetic diversity in the Antarctic toothfish (*Dissostichus mawsoni*) observed with mitochondrial and intron DNA markers. *CCAMLR Science* 12, 43-51.

Stager JC, Johnson TC (2008) The late Pleistocene desiccation of Lake Victoria and the origin of its endemic biota. *Hydrobiologia* 596, 5-16.

Stearns SC (1976) Life-history tactics: a review of the ideas. *Q Rev Biol* 51, 3-45.

*Stepien CA, Murphy DJ, Strange RM (2007) Broad- to fine-scale population genetic patterning in the smallmouth bass *Micropterus dolomieu* across the Laurentian Great

Lakes and beyond: an interplay of behaviour and geography. *Molecular Ecology* 16, 1605-1624.

*Streelman JT, Albertson RC, Kocher TD (2007) Variation in body size and trophic morphology within and among genetically differentiated populations of the cichlid fish, *Metriaclima zebra*, from Lake Malawi. *Freshwater Biology* 52 (3), 525-538.

Streelman JT, Alfaro M, Westneat MW, Bellwood DR, Karl SA (2002) Evolutionary history of the parrotfishes: biogeography, ecomorphology, and comparative diversity. *Evolution* 56, 961-971.

Sturmbauer C (1998) Explosive speciation in cichlid fishes of the African Great Lakes: a dynamic model of adaptive radiation. *Journal of Fish Biology* 53 (Supplement A), 18-36.

Sturmbauer C, Baric S, Salzburger W, Rüber L, Verheyen E (2001) Lake level fluctuations synchronize genetic divergences of cichlid fishes in African lakes. *Mol Biol Evol* 18, 144-154.

Sturmbauer C, Hainz U, Baric S, Verheyen E, Salzburger W (2003) Evolution of the tribe Tropheini from Lake Tanganyika: synchronized explosive speciation producing multiple evolutionary parallelism. *Hydrobiologia* 500, 51-64.

Taberlet P, Fumagalli L, Wust-Saucy A, Cosson J (1998) Comparative phylogeo-graphy and postglacial colonization routes in Europe. *Molecular Ecology* 7, 453-464.

*Taylor MI, Verheyen E (2001) Microsatellite data reveals weak population substructuring in *Copadichromis sp.* 'virginalis kajose', a demersal cichlid from Lake Malawi, Africa. *Journal of Fish Biology* 59, 593-604.

Taylor MS, Hellberg ME (2005) Marine radiations at small geographic scales: speciation in neotropical reef gobies (*Elacatinus*). *Evolution* 59, 374-385.

*Teterina VI, Sukhanova LV, Bogdanov BE, Anoshko PN, Kirilchik SV (2005) Genetic polymorphism of a pelagic fish species, little Baikal oilfish *Comephorus dybowski*, deduced from analysis of microsatellite loci. *Animal Genetics* 41 (7), 750-754.

Thatje S, Hillenbrand CD, Larter R (2005) On the origin of Antarctic marine benthic community structure. *Trends in Ecology and Evolution* 20 (10), 534-540.

*Tinti F, di Nunno C, Guarniero I, Talenti M, Tommasini S, Fabbri E, Picinetti C (2002) Mitochondrial DNA sequence variation suggests the lack of genetic heterogeneity in the Adriatic and Ionian stocks of *Sardina pilchardus*. *Marine Biotechnology* 4, 163-172.

*van Oppen MJ, Turner GF, Rico C, Deutsch JC, Ibrahim KM, Robinson RL, Hewitt GM (1997) Unusually fine-scale genetic structuring found in rapidly speciating Malawi cichlid fishes. *Proc R Soc Lond B Biol Sci* 264, 1803-1812.

*Vasconcellos AV, Vianna P, Paiva PC, Schama R, Solé-Cava A (2008) Genetic and morphometric differences between yellowtail snapper (*Ocyurus chrysurus*, Lutjanidae) populations of the tropical West Atlantic. *Genetics and Molecular Biology* 31, 308-316.

Verheyen E, Salzburger W, Snoeks J, Meyer A (2003) Origin of the superflock of cichlid fishes from Lake Victoria, East Africa. *Science* 300, 325-329.

Veron JEN (1995) *Corals in space and time: biogeography and evolution of the Scleractinia.* Comstock/Cornell, Ithaca, NY.

*Vonlanthen P, Excoffier L, Bittner D, Persat H, Neuenschwander S, Largiadèr CR (2007) Genetic analysis of potential postglacial watershed crossings in Central Europe by the bullhead (*Cottus gobio* L.). *Molecular Ecology* 16, 4572-4584.

Vonlanthen P, Roy D, Hudson AG, Largiader CR, Bittner D, Seehausen O (2009) Divergence along a steep ecological gradient in lake whitefish (*Coregonus* sp.). *J Evol Biol* 22, 498-514.

Wainwright PC, Bellwood DR, Westneat MW, Grubich JR, Hoey AS (2004) A functional morphospace for the skull of labrid fishes: patterns of diversity in a complex biomechanical system. *Biological Journal of the Linnean Society* 82, 1-25.

*Walter RP, Haffner GD, Heath DD (2009) Dispersal and population genetic structure of Telmatherina antoniae, an endemic freshwater Sailfin silverside from Sulawesi, Indonesia. *Journal of Evolutionary Biology* 22 (2), 314-323.

Westneat MW (1997) Phylogenetic relationships of labrid fishes: an analysis of morphological characters. *Am Zool* 37, 198A.

Westneat MW (1999) The living marine resources of the Western Central Pacific: FAO species identification sheets for fishery purposes. Family Labridae. *Food and Agriculture Organization of the United Nations* 6, 3381–3467.

Westneat MW, Alfaro ME (2005) Phylogenetic relationships and evolutionary history of the reef fish family Labridae. *Molecular Phylogenetics and Evolution* 36, 370-390.

White MG (1998) Development, dispersal and recruitment - a paradox for survival among Antarctic fish. In: *Fishes of Antarctica. A biological overview* (eds. di Prisco G, Pisano E, Clarke A). Springer-Verlag, Milano, Italy.

Williams GC (1966) *Adaptation and natural selection. A critique of some current evolutionary thought*. Princeston University Press, Princeton.

Wu C-I (2001) The genic view of the process of speciation. *J Evol Biol* 14, 851-865.

*Wu GCC, Chiang HC, Chen KS (2009) Population structure of albacore (*Thunnus alalunga*) in the Northwestern Pacific Ocean inferred from mitochondrial DNA. *Fisheries Research* 95, 125-131.

*Xiao Y, Takahashi M, Yanagimotot T, Zhang Y, Gao T, Yabe M, Sakurai Y (2008) Genetic variation and population structure of willowy flounder *Tanakius kitaharai* collected from Aomori, Ibaraki and Niigata in Northern Japan. *African Journal of Biotechnology* 7 (21), 3836-3844.

*Zane L, Bargelloni L, Bortolotto E, Papetti C, Simonato M, Varotto V, Patarnello T (2006) Demographic history and population structure of the Antarctic silverfish *Pleuragramma antarcticum*. *Molecular Evolution,* 15 (14), 4499-4511.

In: Phylogeography
Editor: Damien S. Rutgers

ISBN: 978-1-60692-954-4
© 2013 Nova Science Publishers, Inc.

Chapter 2

PHYLOGEOGRAPHY: ITS IMPORTANCE IN INSECT PEST CONTROL

M. D. Ochando, A. Reyes, D. Segura and C. Callejas
Departamento de Genética, Facultad de CC. Biológicas,
Universidad Complutense, Madrid, Spain

1. SUMMARY

Phylogeography involves knowledge of the spatial distribution of related individuals and historical information on the relationship within and among populations and species. The phylogeography of many groups has been studied over recent decades, and this field of knowledge is now becoming important in solving the problems of pest control in agriculture and forestry. An understanding of the nature of the genetic variation within and between pest populations is of paramount importance in the design of pest control programmes and their success – and successful programs are certainly needed since increasing levels of trade and passenger travel, the growth of new plant species in new regions and climate change are all assisting the spread of economically important insect pests.

Molecular genetics is now providing us with new and more sensitive tools for developing appropriate insect control and eradication strategies. Our group is studying the genetic variation of tephritids and whiteflies, both of which are important pests of agricultural and ornamental plants in the Mediterranean region (ecosystems). The information presented here is a summary of some of the results obtained in enzyme electrophoresis (MLEE), abundant soluble protein content, random amplification of polymorphic DNA (RAPD-PCR), intermicrosatellite (ISSR), restriction fragment length polymorphism (RFLP) and mtDNA sequencing analyses. These data document the phylogeographic structure of these taxa's populations, and provide information regarding their bioinvasion and colonisation of new areas, their geographic variation, and gene flow among regions. Such information could be helpful in the taking of pest management decisions, and highlights the need for the coordination of control programs between regional, national and international authorities.

2. The Problem

Insect pests are a growing problem worldwide; increasing levels of trade and passenger travel, the growth of new plant species in new regions and climate change are all assisting the spread of economically important insect pests. These pests cause tremendous harvest and economic losses, including prevention, quarantine, and eradication costs. Globally, the cost of the damage caused by invasive species has been estimated at close to 5% of the world's GDP, and in developing countries, where agriculture accounts for a higher proportion of the GDP, the negative impact of invasive species can be even greater (CABI, http://www.cabi.org).

In the past, synthetic pesticides (insecticides, fungicides and herbicides) seemed to be the solution to pest control and were seen as an integral part of agricultural intensification. The "green revolution" understood pesticides to be essential in improving harvests, and government instruments were made available to help make them accessible to farmers. However, just a few decades later the indiscriminate use, misuse and overuse of pesticides has led to increased resistance on the part of the pests they were meant to kill. Pesticide residues in food have become an important human health concern, and the pollution of the environment by these agents has led to concerns over the health of ecosystems and the loss of biodiversity. People are now realizing that while pesticides can be successful in the short term, they can cause many more problems than they solve in the long term. Pesticide use is now more controlled, with national and international laws establishing strict controls that favour the reduced use of pesticides, and the European Union is strictly controlling the quality of imported fresh food, meaning exporting countries must apply pesticide use controls. Nonetheless, these agents are still employed in huge amounts around the world.

The indiscriminate use of pesticides has required changes be made in plant protection strategies. Indeed, since the mid 1960s the FAO has been advocating Integrated Pest Management (IPM) as the preferred pest control strategy. IPM, as defined by the Dictionary of Biological Control (Coombs and Coombs, 2003), is "a system for controlling pests that is based on the combined use of a range of different methods (e.g., biopesticides, biocontrol agents, mating disruption, trapping and crop rotation, etc.) in order to minimise the use of chemical pesticides". IPM methods try to be more environmentally sensitive in their approach to pest management than other classical methods. IPM programs have been numerous and have been implemented in many developed countries. However, they face more problems in developing countries since they require more than the involvement of farmers, such as field staff from national and local governments and non-governmental institutions. Together these have the job of enhancing ecological awareness, of making evident the need for long term economic benefits, and of promoting environmental and human health safety. In summary, IPMs promote the growth of healthy crops by encouraging natural pest control mechanisms (FAO, http://www.fao.org/) and in so doing try to cause the least possible disruption of agro-ecosystems.

Later on, a derived system, Area-Wide Integrated Pest Management (AW-IPM) seeks to ensure protection from pests over very large regions, and so avoid new invasions. Conventional insect control has been, in general, short-term and small-area in its thinking, with little planning, and has involved the use of simple technology. However, such programs have commonly run into trouble and have required a move to area-wide insect control involving large numbers of producers and crops. The aim of area-wide control is to reduce the pest population within a large target area to a non-economically important level. This is accomplished by attacking the entire insect pest population in the target area (Tan, ed., 2000; Vreysen *et al*., eds., 2007). To increase efficacy, high technology systems that can reduce costs and environmental problems are required.

An important point to address from the beginning in AW-IPM is the selection of the target pest. Many species might be candidates for control, but selection must start with those species that cause the greatest damage and that have the widest distribution, e.g., tephritids such as *Ceratitis capitata* and *Bactrocera oleae* etc. As has been pointed out, IPM is a defensive procedure practised from a field point of view basis, but now, for AW-IPM to have the best chances of success, information on the structure and dynamics of populations and on the phylogeography of those populations is necessary (Cox, 2007).

Back in 1964, DeBach defined Biological Control (BC) as "...the action of parasites, predators or pathogens in maintaining another organism's population density at a lower average than would occur in their absence". Nowadays, BC is considered part of IPM and is becoming more popular, in part because of the surge in ecological agriculture and the increasing demand for its products. These days the definition has changed somewhat to reflect a more applied concept and has become "the use of predatory and parasitic insect species (termed natural enemies or beneficials), or natural products consisting of or derived from microorganisms, against pests and disease of crops" (Coombs and Coombs, 2003). For a good review of Biological Control see Bellows and Fisher (1999). However it should not be forgotten that, in many cases, chemical pesticides may also be required for the pest density to be brought a level at which BC is feasible.

The ultimate aim of BC is to maintain pest populations at a low level or eradicate them, thus reducing the risks of survival of sources of later reinfestation. However, BC requires more complete and intensive management and planning, the training of personnel, and it can take more time to achieve results. Some major successes has been achieved with BC, but the outcome of its use is normally far from predictable. Less than 30% of all attempts to achieve the control of pests via the introduction of its natural enemies are successful (Greathead and Greathead, 1992; Unruh and Woolley, 1999).

Currently, IPM, AW-IPM and BC are all implemented by governments and international organizations (e.g., the FAO, IOBC, International Organization of Biological Control, CABI, the Centre for Agriculture and Biosciences International [formerly the Commonwealth Agricultural Bureaux International]), and different governmental and non-governmental authorities are working to make farmers and the public aware of its possibilities, organizing meetings to discuss its use, and developing research projects, etc. Such is the case of the International Organization of Biological Control (IOBC, which is divided into a number of working groups and regional sections) which "promotes the use of sustainable, environmentally safe, economically feasible and socially acceptable control methods of pests and diseases of agricultural and forestry crops", and encourages collaboration in the development and promotion of biological and integrated production systems. The IOBC trains people in and informs people about biological methods of control, as well as the use of chemicals, within an IPM context. It also produces guidelines for the integrated production of crops, develops and standardises methods of testing the effects of pesticides on beneficial species, and organises scientific meetings and research on insect pests (IOBC: http://www.iobc-wprs.org/). Phylogenetic studies are now more commonly reported in such meetings.

3. THE CHALLENGE

The EU is a major player in global agricultural trade; indeed, it is the largest importer and the second largest exporter of foodstuffs, it plays a leading role in establishing global trade agreements via the World Trade Organisation (WTO) and the European Commission of Agricultural and Rural Development (via the Common Agricultural Policy [CAP]), and it promotes sustainable agriculture in a global environment. It should be remembered that 90% of the land within the EU is either farmland or forestry. Farmers still receive subsidies, but in compensation they have to respect environmental safety, food safety and phytosanitary and animal welfare standards. The CAP not only ensures standards for EU farmers, it improves the quality of Europe's food (helping to guarantee food safety) and ensures that the environment is protected for future generations (http://ec.europa.eu/agriculture).

The European Commission is working on a strategy to reduce the impact of pesticides on human health and the environment. In fact, the last assessment on the European environment (The fourth assessment, 2007) highlights that "the historic impact of agriculture on landscapes and biodiversity was positive, but modern, intensive agriculture is often a threat to biodiversity. Agriculture has a negative influence the on environment through its use and pollution of resources such as air, water and soil". Fortunately, pesticide use appears to have been decreasing throughout the region since 1990, and the trend is towards the complete elimination of these chemicals.

While authorities are legislating for a more rational and safer use of pesticides, trying to enhance the development and current acceptance of IPM and BC, the conviction exists that better scientific knowledge of insect pests and their natural enemies will lead to more effective biological control. Indeed, agricultural associations are now demanding the EU legislate on a scientific basis. In this regard, molecular methods may provide us new characters of study to diversify our knowledge of the phylogenetic relationships of pests, to identify different biotypes and better understand their ecology and population structures, etc., and in so doing contribute towards better biological control and better legislation. In other words, from research to implementation.

4. THE TOOLS: BIOGEOGRAPHY ANDMOLECULAR GENETICS

Phylogeography involves knowledge of the spatial distribution of related individuals and historical information on the relationship within and among populations and species (Avise, 1994, 2000; Lomolino *et al.*, 2006). The phylogeography of many groups has been studied in recent decades, but only recently has this field of knowledge started to become important in the study of insect pests in agriculture, ornamental plants and forestry. Detailed knowledge of the biology, genetic structure and geographical variability of a given pest species is a prerequisite in planning strategies for its quarantine, control or eradication (Roderick and Navajas, 2003). For example, the reconstruction of the histories of populations can be important in identifying the natural enemies of pests that can be used in biological control. Further, the identification of pathways of anthropogenically mediated introductions can assist in international efforts to limit the spread of non-indigenous pests. Different insect pest studies have demonstrated the value of knowledge on population genetics in pest management (Villablanca *et al.*, 1998; Gasperi *et al.* 2002; Meixner *et al.*, 2002; Ochando *et al.*, 2003a, b, etc.).

The role of molecular genetics technologies in studies related to population structure and the dynamics of insect pest species has increased rapidly during the last two decades. Rapid improvements in resolution, reproducibility, time, costs and standardization, plus recognition from insect control managers and authorities regarding the importance of such studies, is leading to the general acceptance that phylogenetic knowledge is a cornerstone in our fight against insect pests.

DNA methodologies in general, and those based on the polymerase chain reaction (PCR) in particular, are currently being used to answer a range of questions and are contributing significantly to our knowledge of population structures and dynamics, genetic mapping and phylogeny etc. (Loxdale and Lushai, 1998; Avise, 2003, 2004; Severson *et al.*, 2001; Heckel, 2003; Mendelson and Shaw 2005; Behura, 2006). They are also supplying more applied knowledge on insect/plant/pathogen interactions, insecticide resistance, mating behaviour related to sterile insect technique (SIT), and on the predators and parasites of pest species, etc. The use of both kind, nuclear and mitochondrial, markers have contributed to advances in our knowledge, and studies on amplified fragment length polymorphism (AFLP), random amplified polymorphic DNA (RAPD) and microsatellites, and the use of many others types of PCR technology (S-SAP, SNP, EPIC etc.), are slowly becoming popular tools for tackling insect pest problems (for a review of the use of molecular markers in insect studies see Behura, 2006). Advances in the inference of phylogenetic relationships from molecular data, however, require the use of appropriate statistical tools, and advances are also significant in this way (Swofford *et al.*, 1996; Nei and Kumar, 2000; Felsenstein, 2004).

Analysis of molecular data in a phylogenetic context requires that one be aware of the particular properties of the different types of data and of the different analytical approaches to data analysis. As have been marked by Unruh and Woolley (1999), three questions must be asked when one is contemplating a phylogenetic study involving molecular markers. The first one is about the rate of evolution of the marker, is it a rate appropriate for the biological system under study?. One of the reasons that mtDNA has been used so successfully in many studies of infraspecific phylogeography is that restriction endonucleases generate useful and informative variation at the level of local populations. Second, are we making the comparisons between homologous features in different taxa? do we know sufficiently the source of variation of the used marker?. And third, are our methods of analysis sensitive enough to detect variation in rates of evolution among different marker systems, or between different taxa when using a single marker system?.

Phylogenetic methods have several distinct advantages. Certainly they provide a simple and rigorous context in which to directly compare information from various sources e.g., different sequences of DNA and types (from a selective point of view) of DNA fragments, allozymes and morphology. Another advantage is that such information can provide direct evidence supporting the existence of particular clades (groups or lineages).

In sum, the biogeographic information obtained through the use of these molecular technologies is probably now one of our most powerful tools in the eventual control of insect pests.

5. SPECIFIC QUESTIONS

The agricultural, forestry and ornamental plants importance of insect pests highlights the need to understand pest population structures and dynamics. Phylogeographic genetics is helping to answer basic questions regarding bioinvasions, the geographic sources of invasions, population genetic structures, gene flow, host/geographic biotypes and colonisation routes etc. This chapter reports some of the results (partly already published) obtained by our group in these areas regarding pests of Spain and the Mediterranean Basin in general. The overall aim of our research was to use DNA marker methodologies to study the phylogeography, geographic population structure, gene flow, molecular systematic and phylogenetics of insect pests, and to make known the importance of this kind of work in the outcome of pest control management actions.

6. BIOINVASIONS: WHITEFLIES IN THE CANARY ISLANDS

The invasion of an area by an exotic species could be a unique event or the outcome of waves of re-introduction?. Can the origin of the invader be determined?

The increasing level of trade, the cultivation of plant species in new regions and climate change may all be significant aspects related to the invasion a territory by exotic pests. Spain is the gateway between Europe and Africa, which lies just 14 km away across the Straits of Gibraltar. Spain's biodiversity is the highest in Europe – but it is also a part of the continent likely to be most affected by climate change. Further, it is the most important point of trade and travel between Europe and Central and South America. Together, these factors leave Spain particularly vulnerable to bioinvasions. Some recent examples include the arrival of new and more pathogenic biotypes of the whitefly *Bemisia tabaci* in the country's greenhouses, and the appearance –now or in a short time expected- of *Bactrocera zonata*. In addition, the European Food Security Agency of (EFSA) has confirmed that the pest control measures applied by the EU to citrus fruits imported from South Africa are insufficient, with the consequent risk of the introduction of the fungus *Guignardia citricarpa* (the causal agent of black spot). Moreover, in the Mediterranean region of Spain, three other exotic pests have been detected over the last two years. Tougher controls are therefore required - controls that need to be based on better scientific knowledge. Phylogeographic information could be of paramount importance in this respect.

The whitefly *Aleurodicus dispersus* (Russell 1965, Hemiptera, Aleyrodidae) is a highly polyphagous, haplodiploid species that has been recorded on about 100 species of plants belonging to nearly 30 families, including many ornamental, vegetable and fruit crops (Waterhouse and Norris, 1989). This species, native to the Caribbean region, was first recorded in the Canary Islands in 1965 on *Schinus terebinthifolius*. Since then, it has spread throughout the archipelago (Hernández-Suarez *et al.*, 1997; Beitia, 1998; Martin *et al.,* 2000), and since the 1990s it has been an important pest on ornamental and tropical crops. The nature of the invasion process and the geographic source of the original invading population were questions to which control managers needed answers – answers that the phylogeographic studies undertaken by our group helped provide (Callejas *et al.*, 2005).

To investigate recent bioinvasions of exotic species, markers revealing the variation among recently diverged populations are needed. We decided to use RAPD markers. The Random Amplified Polymorphic DNA technique (Williams *et al.* 1990; Welch and McClelland, 1990) involves the amplification of random polymorphic segments of genomic DNA using single primers of arbitrary nucleotide sequence. Like any other genetic marker, RAPD markers have some limitations, including limited reproducibility and marker dominance. Among the DNA fingerprinting techniques, however, RAPD requires the least economic input, the smallest amount of laboratory equipment and labour, its usefulness in insect population studies is well known, and most importantly, RAPD markers show a very high degree of variability among samples at the infraspecific level. RAPD-PCR was therefore used to study seven samples of *A. dispersus* from different hosts on different islands of the Canary group (Figure 1). Fifty adults from each population were analysed, along with 14 pupae from Costa Rica, which were used as an outgroup.

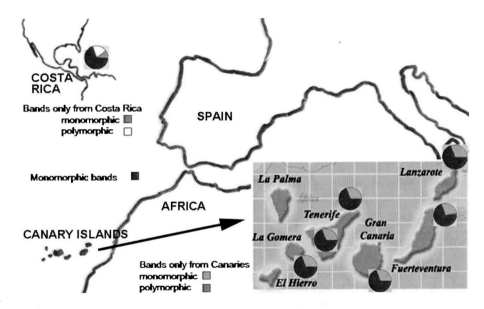

Figure 1. Collection sites and frequencies and distribution of monomorphic and polymorphic RAPD bands for populations of *A. dispersus* from the Canaries and Costa Rica.

Genomic DNA was extracted according to our own protocol based on that of Higuchi (1989) with some modifications. Six primers - A03, A13, B08, C08, F06 and F08 - (Operon technologies, Alameda, USA) were used. The amplification reactions were performed according to Williams *et al.* (1990) with minor modifications. The thermocycler program used was: preheating at 94°C for 5 min, 45 cycles of amplification (1 min at 94°C, 1 min at 36°C, 6 min at 72°C) and a final extension step of 6 min at 72°C. Along with a standard molecular weight marker (100 bp Ladder Plus, MBI Fermentas) the PCR amplification products were loaded onto 2.0% agarose gels in a buffer solution (1X TAE) containing ethidium bromide (0.5 µg/ml). All reactions were performed following a strict protocol with standardised conditions, repeating each amplification reaction at least twice. All the amplification products obtained were reproducible and consistent. Figure 2 shows an example of the RAPD profiles obtained with primer A03.

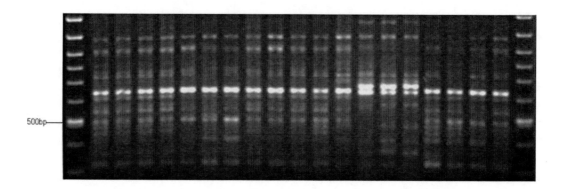

Figure 2. RAPD profiles of the *A. dispersus* flies analyzed with primer A03. First and last lanes contain a 100bp ladder molecular weight marker and the remaining correspond to specimens from different populations.

A total of 68 bands were scored, their size ranging from 240 to 1400 bp. No differences in RAPD patterns were found among the samples from the different Canary islands, except for one exclusive band present in just one fly from Lanzarote (Figure 1).

Unexpectedly, the number of generations elapsed from the first detection of the pest in the Canary Islands (9-12 per year, Hernández-Suarez, 1999) seems not to have been enough to generate variability or to provide evidence of possible selection effects. The founder effect therefore appears to have been very strong. Haplodiploid species may commonly show reduced genetic variability compared to those in which both sexes are diploid; in the haploid sex all loci would be subject to selection.

Our results show there to be no genetic differences in *A. dispersus* inhabiting the different islands of the Canary archipelago. Neither were any differences observed relating to geographic origin, host/plant relationship or year of sampling. This very low level of genetic variation, with all populations showing the same DNA bands, supports the hypothesis of a single colonisation event by a small number of *A. dispersus* whiteflies followed by recent dispersion from the introduction point.

The results for the Costa Rican outgroup flies were quite different from those of the Canary Island populations. Thirty six of the total 68 bands scored (53%) showed fixed differences between the samples from the Canary Islands and Costa Rica. 'Regional' diagnostic bands, i.e, bands of DNA present in all whiteflies from the Canary Islands but absent in those from the outgroup and *vice versa* were also found: 11 in the Costa Rican whiteflies (including five that were polymorphic) and 15 in those from the Canary Islands. Thus, the flies of these two regions are quite well differentiated. Costa Rica is therefore not the source of the Canary Islands infestation.

In summary, the results of these RAPD phylogeographic studies suggest that the colonisation of the Canary Islands by *A. dispersus* began with a single colonisation event followed by dispersion, and that these invaders did not come from Costa Rica.

7. COLONISATION PATTERNS: THE IBERIAN PENINSULA IN THE EXPANSION HISTORY OF THE MEDFLY

Can the colonisation process of a pest that has been established in a region for a long time be known? Can origin and expansion routes of such a pest be determined?

Intraspecific historical phylogeography - the study of the geographic distribution of a genealogical lineage (Avise *et al.*, 1987; Avise, 1991a, b, 2000) - was introduced at the end of 1970s, mostly involving mtDNA studies (especially restriction fragment length polymorphism [RFLP] studies). This technique was much more powerful and informative than those previously used, such as allozyme studies or even the measurement of nuclear sequence variation. The maternal inheritance of mtDNA, its rate of evolution, its lack of recombination and introns, its extensive polymorphism and the relative ease of its purification offer clear advantages in intraspecific phylogeography studies (Avise, 1994; Swofford *et al.*, 1996; Unruh and Woolley, 1999). Indeed, mtDNA markers have been among the most useful in population and phylogeographic analyses of all species (Avise, 1986; Hillis *et al.*, 1996; Zhang and Hewitt, 1997; Behura, 2006).

Along with MLEE, abundant soluble protein, RAPD-PCR and ISSR techniques, we used RFLP to study the colonisation history of *C. capitata* in the Iberian Peninsula. From a phylogeographic point of view, and for determining the colonisation route followed by the pest, the results shown below are some of the most important obtained.

The family Tephritidae (Tephritidae, Diptera), with more than 4000 fly species, is probably one of the most economically important of all the Diptera. The majority of its species are fruit pests, and the Mediterranean fruit fly, *Ceratitis capitata* (Wiedemann) (Diptera: Tephritidae) is among the world's most destructive and economically devastating pest species (Figure 3). It is responsible for direct economic losses in fruit production, and is the focus of considerable and costly detection and eradication programs in all countries where it is found (Dowel and Krass, 1992; Bohonak *et al.*, 2001; Silva *et al.*, 2003; Meixner *et al.*, 2002; Ochando *et al.*, 2007; Malacrida *et al.*, 2007; Aluja and Mangan, 2008). Over the last 150/200 years, the medfly has expanded rapidly via its own power of dispersal and via human-mediated transport from its putative source area in Central Africa (Hagen *et al.*, 1981) to almost all regions with temperate or tropical climates (the Mediterranean region, South Africa, Central and South America, and even Australia) (Fletcher, 1989). It has even recently been detected in North America. The original host of the species was *Argaria spinosa* (L.), but the medfly now infests more than 250 species and varieties of agriculturally important plants (Fimiani, 1989). It is suspected that the Iberian Peninsula has played an important role in the spread of *C. capitata* to the Mediterranean region (Hagen *et al.*, 1981) and possibly to some regions of America. Genetic studies of wild Spanish populations of *C. capitata* may help to reveal its pattern of invasion and, subsequently, assist in designing strategies for its control and eradication.

Over the last 10 years a number of authors have attempted to resolve the fine geographical scale of medfly invasions, and to determine the genetic structure of its populations using different kinds of genetic markers (MLEE: Reyes and Ochando, 1994; Baruffi *et al.*, 1995; Malacrida *et al.*, 1998; Ochando *et al.*, 2003a; microsatellites: Bonizzoni *et al.*, 2000, 2001, 2004; Meixner *et al.*, 2002; RAPD: Haymer and McInnis, 1994; Baruffi *et al.*, 1995; Reyes and Ochando, 1998; Gasperi *et al.*, 2002; intron loci: Gomulski *et al.*, 1998;

M. D. Ochando, A. Reyes, D. Segura et al.

Villablanca *et al.*, 1998; Davies *et al.*, 1999; He and Haymer, 1999; RFLP of mtDNA: Silva *et al.*, 2003; Reyes and Ochando, 2004, etc.).

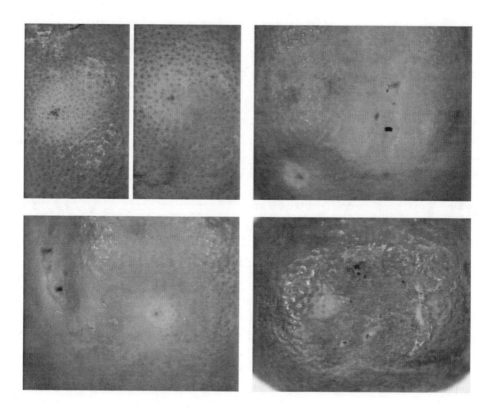

Figure 3. Infested citrus fruits by *Ceratitis capitata*.

However, as Davies *et al.* (1999) have stated "*... genetic analysis...should begin with mtDNA...*". We used RFLP of mtDNA to study the variation of Spanish populations of *C. capitata* (Reyes and Ochando, 1998b, 2004). The aim of the work was to provide information about the phylogeographic relationships of medfly populations in this region, and the colonisation route taken across the northern Mediterranean.

Flies from different parts of Spain were collected by harvesting infested fruit and allowing the larvae to pupate in the laboratory. Twenty isofemale lines survived under laboratory conditions during the experiment: five from a population from central Spain (40°27'N 3°49'W, about 600 km north of the Straits of Gibraltar; known as population CENTRE), five from a population from eastern Spain (39°26'N 1°10'W, about 70 km from the Mediterranean coast and 700 km northeast of the Straits of Gibraltar; known as population EAST), and 10 derived from a population from southern Spain (36°30'N 5°20'W, about 70 km north of the Straits of Gibraltar; known as population SOUTH). Mitochondrial DNA was obtained according to Afonso *et al.* (1988) with minor modifications. RFLP was studied using 22 restriction endonucleases, 17 of which (*Asp* 718, *Bam*H I, *Bcl* I, *Bst*E II, *Cla* I, *Dra* I, *Eco*R I, *Eco*R V, *Hin*d III, *Hpa* I, *Pst* I, *Pvu* II, *Sac* I, *Sal* I, *Sma* I, *Xba* I and *Xho* I) recognized 6 bp sequences, and five of which (*Cfo* I, *Hae* III, *Hin*f I, *Hpa* II and *Rsa* I) recognized 4 bp sequences. The restriction fragments obtained were resolved in 0.8-1.5%

agarose gels in the presence of TAE buffer containing ethidium bromide (0.5µg/µl). Lambda phage digested with *Hin*d III or *Bst*E II was used as a molecular marker.

Ten of these endonucleases (*Bcl* I, *Eco*R I, *Eco*R V, *Hin*d III, *Hpa* II, *Pvu* II, *Rsa* I, *Sac* I, *Xba* I and *Xho* I) yielded the same pattern for all the isofemale lines, five did not cut the *C. capitata* mtDNA (*Cla* I, *Hpa* I, *Pst* I, *Sal* I and *Sma* I), and the remaining seven enzymes (*Asp* 718, *Bam*H I, *Bst*E II, *Cfo* I, *Dra* I, *Hae* III and *Hin*f I) revealed RFLP. A total of 65 mtDNA restriction sites seen in the 20 isofemale strains of *C. capitata*; 59 (90.8%) were the same for all strains while the other six (9.2%) were polymorphic (Figure 4).

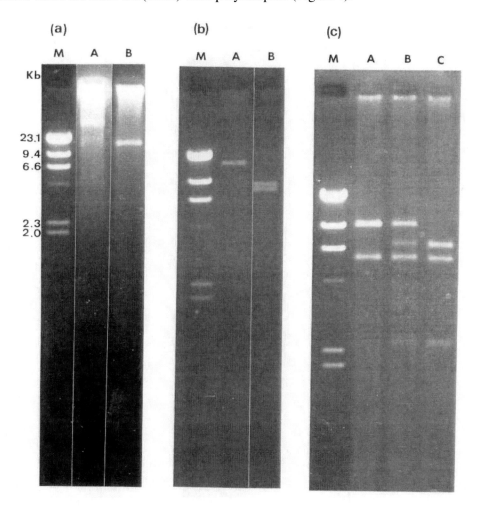

Figure 4. Restriction fragment length polymorphism profiles with restriction endonucleases *Asp* 718 (a), *Bst*E II (b) and *Hae* III (c) of *Ceratitis capitata* specimens. Molecular weight marker (M) corresponds to lambda phage cut with *Hin*d III.

The combination of single patterns resulted in nine composite patterns or haplotypes, numbered I to IX. Based on a maximum parsimony network (see Reyes and Ochando, 2004, for a detailed explanation of the unrooted tree), haplotypes II and VII were found to be in central positions. Haplotypes VII and VIII were the only two present in all three Spanish populations, while haplotypes I to VI were present only in population SOUTH, and haplotype

IX was present only in population CENTRE. Thus, haplotype VII can be deemed the ancestral haplotype in Spain.

As mentioned above, haplotypes I to VI and IX were found only in single populations - SOUTH and CENTRE respectively. This suggests that they appeared after the colonisation of these areas. Moreover, the haplotypes present in more than one population (VII and VIII) appear with different frequencies (Figure 5). All the haplotypes (except one) were present only in population SOUTH. Maximum likelihood analysis (Nei and Li, 1979; Nei and Tajima, 1981) showed the nucleotide diversity to be highest in population SOUTH (0.30%), followed by CENTRE (0.24%), and finally by EAST (0.06%).

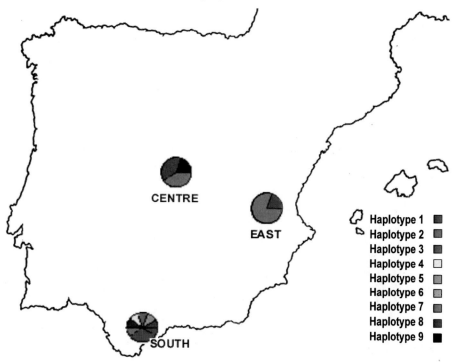

CENTRE

EAST

Haplotype 1
Haplotype 2
Haplotype 3
Haplotype 4
Haplotype 5
Haplotype 6
Haplotype 7
Haplotype 8
Haplotype 9

SOUTH

Figure 5. Population sampling sites and mtDNA haplotypes frequencies and distribution in the three populations of *Ceratitis capitata* analysed.

The colonisation of Spain by this pest is thought to have taken place via the Straits of Gibraltar, followed by its dispersion to more northerly regions (Hagen *et al.*, 1981). Accordingly, a decreasing level of variability from the source area towards the areas more recently colonised should be detected. Indeed, the highest value of nucleotide diversity was found in population SOUTH (0.30%), which is geographically very close to the Straits of Gibraltar (about 70 km). Populations CENTRE and EAST had lower nucleotide diversity values (0.24% and 0.06% respectively). These results are in agreement with those obtained for the same populations when using molecular markers such as isozymes, when using RAPD-PCR (Reyes, 1995), or when examining the content of soluble proteins (Reyes and Ochando, 1998), and with those obtained in other Spanish populations of this species (Reyes and Ochando, 1994).

Medfly populations can be divided into three main categories according to their colonisation pattern: ancestral, ancient and new populations (Malacrida *et al.*, 1992), corresponding to populations from Africa, the Mediterranean Basin and America respectively. The question arises as to whether results from analyses involving the mitochondrial restriction sites in flies from these different regions are in agreement with the proposed colonisation process of this pest. In American populations, only one haplotype per geographical area has been found. In the case of Spanish populations, up to nine different haplotypes have been described, irrespective of sample size. The low degree of genetic variability in American populations (Sheppard *et al.*, 1992; McPheron *et al.*, 1994; Gasparich *et al.*, 1995, 1997; Steck *et al.*, 1996; Meixner *et al.*, 2002) suggests the recent colonisation of America by African populations - both the African and American populations share a haplotype. African haplotypes are not seen, however, in Mediterranean populations. Although most Spanish haplotypes differ from the African haplotypes (Sheppard *et al.*, 1992; Gasparich *et al.*, 1997) by only one mutational step, indicating a possibly direct African origin, the large number of Spanish haplotypes would appear to indicate that the colonisation process is not as recent as in America. Haplotypes from Greece are not directly related to African ones but to Spanish haplotypes, suggesting that they might be derived from Spanish populations. However, this should be interpreted with caution since only one laboratory population from Greece has been analysed (Kourti, 1997). Overall, these findings are substantially in agreement with those obtained with other genetics markers and with the historical reports of movements of this pest (see below).

Isozyme and microsatellites analyses performed on African, American and Mediterranean populations (Huettel *et al.*, 1980; Loukas, 1989; Gasperi *et al.*, 1991; Malacrida *et al.*, 1992, 1998, 2007; Reyes and Ochando, 1994, 1998; Baruffi *et al.*, 1995; Bonizzoni *et al.*, 2000, 2001, 2004; Meixner *et al.*, 2002; Ochando *et al.*, 2003a) have also revealed the greatest genetic variability (assessed by the proportion of polymorphic loci, the mean number of alleles per locus, and the average heterozygosity) to be shown by the populations of Africa, followed by those of the Mediterranean and finally those of America. Among the Mediterranean populations, those of Spain seem to show higher variability than those of Italy, followed by the Greek populations. The results of such macrogeographic analyses appear to be in agreement with one another whatever the molecular marker used. However, from a microgeographic point of view the data are not always so clear. For example, RAPD studies on Spanish populations of *C. capitata* show no clear quantitative nor distribution trends (Reyes, 1995). The explanation may lie in the high genetic flow among regions and the fact that consecutive generations of the fly need to feed on the fruit available at the moment. "Generalist" alleles are therefore required rather than "specialist" alleles that would adapt them to a specific kind of fruit. The non-existence of host biotypes supports such an interpretation (Ochando *et al.*, 2003b)

In summary, the results obtained in mtDNA, isozyme, microsatellite, intron loci and RAPD analyses suggest that *C. capitata* has moved from its source area in Africa to Spain, across the Straits of Gibraltar, probably followed by eastward movements into other northern Mediterranean countries. With respect to the American populations, the low degree of variation (both in mtDNA and isozymes) and the results of intron loci studies (Villablanca *et al.*, 1998; He and Haymer, 1999; Davies *et al.*, 1999) seem to indicate an affinity of these populations with those of Africa - perhaps the result of a recent colonisation event directly from the source area. This hypothesis is in agreement with the dates on which the pest was first noticed in different countries. It was first reported as a pest in Spain in 1842 (De Breme, 1842 cited in Fimiani, 1989), in Italy in 1863 (Martelli, 1910 cited in Fimiani, 1989) and in

Greece in 1915 (Papageorgiou, 1915 cited in Fimiani, 1989). It was then noticed in Argentina in 1905 (Gallo *et al.*, 1970) and in Hawaii in 1910 (Compere, 1912 cited in Headrick and Goeden, 1996). In 1975 it arrived in California (Carey, 1991), and in or before 1955 the medfly successfully established itself in Central America (Sheppard *et al.*, 1992). The progression of these dates is highly concordant with the data obtained with molecular markers.

Notwithstanding, there are other processes besides colonisation that could also influence the degree and/or kind of differentiation seen in the present populations: gene flow and selection. The existence of significant levels of gene flow between populations might limit the geographical differentiation seen between them, even when there is little or no selection. Trade, especially from the south and east to the centre of Spain is extensive, and human mediated movement of the pest between these regions should not be neglected.

In conclusion, the analysis of mtDNA variation in Spanish populations of *C. capitata* revealed them to show low to moderate nucleotide diversity, probably due to the "relatively" recent colonisation (less than two centuries) of Spain by this pest. It would seem, however, that Spanish populations have played an important role in the colonisation of the northern Mediterranean region. The colonisation of America by this species seems to have taken place later than the invasion of Spain and by a different route, probably directly from Africa. More information needs to be collected on *C. capitata* in Spain, not only through "traditional" RFLP analysis, but through a combination with other methods such as intron and ISSR analysis (this is now underway at our laboratory). This could provide more information on levels and patterns of polymorphism, which would be useful in the study of re-invasions and very recently colonised areas.

8. POPULATION STRUCTURE: THE OLIVE FLY IN THE MEDITERRANEAN BASIN

Certain questions arise when considering insect pests with a wide range of distribution that have been established for a long time. Have they differentiated geographically? Is gene flow significant in the prevention of differentiation? Are there different selective pressures at work in different geographic areas?

The olive fruit fly, *Bactrocera oleae* (Gmelin), is a major olive crop pest. Its larvae are monophagous, feeding exclusively on olive fruits (see Figure 6). Crop losses include reduced harvests, reduced oil contents and reduced quality. In the Mediterranean basin, where 98% of the world's cultivated olive trees are found, production losses can reach more than 30%. Olive tree cultivation accounts for some 3.37% of the total agricultural production of the European Union (EU). Spain is the foremost olive oil-producing country in the world, followed by Italy and Greece (data from the FAO, 2004; http://faostat.fao.org/faostat).

The olive fruit fly is widespread throughout the Mediterranean and Middle East, and records of infestations go back some 2300 years (Ruiz, 1948). The pest is also found along the east coast and in the south of Africa, in India and Pakistan, and it was first detected in California in 1998 (Rice *et al.*, 2003). Olive fly researchers generally agree that this insect can survive and develop in any area of the world where olive trees - wild or cultivated - grow (Rice, 2000). Its control relies mainly on chemical treatments, sometimes applied over vast areas by aircraft, with the subsequent ecological and toxicological side effects such practices entail (Alberola *et al.*, 1999).

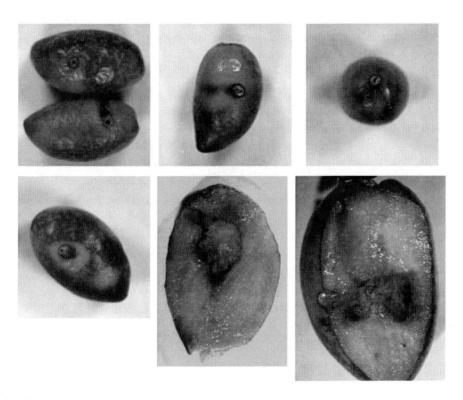

Figure 6. Infested olive fruits by *Bactrocera oleae*.

Given the economic importance of this pest, our knowledge of the olive fly is relatively extensive (see Bush and Kitto, 1979; Zouros and Loukas, 1989; Robinson and Hooper, eds., 1989; Ochando *et al.*, 1994; Barranco *et al.*, eds., 2004), but phylogeographic information is lacking; indeed, only a few recent reports exist (Callejas *et al.*, 1998; Ochando and Reyes, 2000; Ochando *et al.*, 2003a; Nardi *et al.*, 2005; Augustinus *et al.*, 2005). However, the efficient control of this pest requires information on its population structure, its patterns of colonisation, and the origin and spread of invading populations be known. Our group has published several papers on the genetic structure of the populations of the olive fly, mostly from the Mediterranean. Some of the results are summarized below.

In one study, 18 olive fly populations were examined, 13 covering the total range of the pest in the Iberian Peninsula (SP-1, SP-2,....SP-13 and POR), plus one each from Italy (ITA), Greece (GRE), Tunisia (TUN) and Israel (ISR) and California (USA). In all cases (except for the American population), 20 individuals per population were analysed through RAPD-PCR technique. The genomic DNA from individual flies was extracted according to Reyes *et al.* (1997), and DNA amplifications performed according to Williams *et al.* (1990) with minor modifications. Seven arbitrary sequence oligonucleotides (A-02, A-07, A-17, C-05, C-06, C-11 and C-18) from Operon Technologies (Alameda, CA, USA) were used in amplifications performed in an M.J. Research PT-100 thermocycler. The reaction conditions were as follows: preheating to 94° for 5 min, followed by 45 amplification cycles of 1 min at 94°C, 1 min at 36°C and 6 min at 72°C, and a final extension step at 72°C for 6 min. Each amplification reaction was performed at least twice: the results were consistently reproducible. The amplification products were separated according to their molecular size by electrophoresis in 2% agarose gels in the presence of TAE buffer (40 mM Tris-Acetate, 1mM EDTA pH 8.0) and ethidium bromide. A 100 bp ladder marker was used as a molecular size standard.

In general, the polymorphism detected for the olive fly is higher than that reported in RAPD studies of other insects (see De Sousa *et al.*, 1999; Lin *et al.*, 1999; Zitoudi *et al.*, 2001; Ochando *et al.*, 2003a). In our study a total of 115 bands were obtained, 98 of which were polymorphic and 17 monomorphic, and a high level of polymorphism was seen (mean 63%; range 51-70%) (Figure 7). The population diversity, as measured by Shannon's diversity index (H), ranged from 3.93 to 5.28. The literature (Zouros and Loukas, 1989; Ochando *et al.*, 2003a; Nardi *et al.*, 2005; Augustinus *et al.*, 2005) suggests high genetic variability to be characteristic of the species.

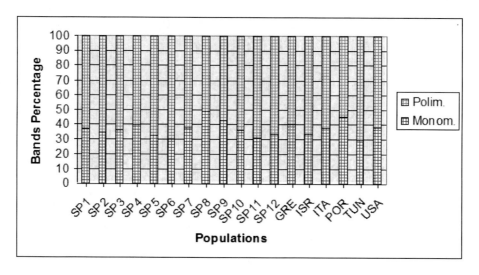

Figure 7. Percentage of monomorphic and polymorphic bands for each population of *B. oleae* sampled, indicated on the figure with different colours.

According to some authors a positive correlation is to be expected between the degree of environmental diversity of a species and its degree of genetic variability, and the potential for ecological heterogeneity to promote genetic diversity, and perhaps divergence, has been proposed (Abrahamson and Weis, 1997; Downie *et al.*, 2001). However, this does not seem to be the case for *B. oleae*. Indeed, comparisons with the information available for other Tephritidae underscores the idea that olive fly populations keep great genetic variation (Yong, 1992; Kourti, 2004; Callejas and Ochando, 2004).

The high genetic variability of *B. oleae* populations is probably due to their large effective size. Olive groves cover wide expanses of territory; they can therefore maintain high population densities. Further, the species became established in the Mediterranean a long time ago. It is thought that it arrived in Europe more than two thousand years ago with the introduction of the olive tree from Western Asia and Africa by the Phoenicians (Ruiz, 1948).

The Californian population also showed high variability (polymorphism value = 62 and the Shannon index: 3.93), which is of the same order as that seen in its European counterparts. These data indicate that this population is most likely the descendant of Mediterranean colonisers (as indicated by Nardi *et al.*, 2005) with a high degree of polymorphism, or that it has been established in America for some time.

However, all the primers used detected lower levels of genetic differentiation among the populations than within them. As much as 86% of the total diversity was attributable to diversity within populations, and just 14% to differences among populations. Similarly, AMOVA analyses showed that nearly all the total genetic variation to be maintained within populations (from 85.07 to 92.28% depending on the analysis). A random permutational test revealed that these variance components were all significant ($p<0.001$). For a detailed explanation of these data see Segura *et al.* (2007, 2008). These results agree with previous data recorded for this species (Zouros and Loukas, 1989; Ochando *et al.*, 1994; Callejas *et al.*, 1998), especially with the data on microsatellites and mitochondrial sequences reported by Nardi *et al.* (2005). Augustinus *et al.* (2005) reported the variation within populations to be 96.11% and the genetic distances between populations to be of the same order as in our work (except for their Cyprus samples) – although these authors draw different conclusions.

Gene flow must be responsible for the uniformity seen among the northern Mediterranean populations of the olive fly (Spanish populations plus Italian, Greek and even Israeli population). The existence of small and isolated populations would lead to divergence between populations and homogeneity within them. Conversely, the presence of large, interconnected populations would result in less interpopulational differentiation and greater diversity within these populations (Lin *et al.*, 1999). Different authors have reported adult olive fly movements ranging from 200 m in the presence of olive hosts, to as much as 4000 m if hosts need to be searched out. Indeed, dispersals of up to 10 km have been reported over open water in the Mediterranean (Rice, 2000). The passive transport of olive flies associated with human activities (such as transport and new plantations of olive trees) must be considered as well. An effective migration rate (Nm) of 1 is sufficient to prevent genetic differentiation among populations (Wright, 1931; Maruyama, 1970, 1972). The gene flow estimated for the Mediterranean populations in our work was more than 4, indicating that this may be an important factor influencing the genetic structure of *B. oleae* in this region where large populations have long been established.

The UPGM dendrogram (Figure 8) shows the relationships among the 18 populations of *B. oleae* analysed in this study. The bootstrap values were generally low (except for the first branching), supporting the idea that the majority of these populations are genetically so similar that they are difficult to separate. Notwithstanding, both the dendrogram and PCA analysis (Figure 8 and Figure 9) show the most southerly of the Mediterranean populations - the African population (TUN) – to differ significantly from the remaining populations. The American (USA) population at the next levels of branching, form a group separated from the rest of the populations. Augustinus *et al.* (2005) reported the existence of subpopulations in the Mediterranean. However, in our case this conclusion is not statistically supported; the Italian, Greek, Israeli and Iberian populations cluster together. These results generally agree with those of Nardi *et al.* (2005) who used others markers (microsatellites and mtDNA sequences); these authors also found two genetics groups, one African (Eastern Africa) and other European (including American populations). In the present case, all the northern Mediterranean populations clustered together. When the dendrogram was produced for the

Iberian populations alone, no clear clustering pattern was observed. In the Iberian Peninsula, olive groves cover huge expanses of territory. This, along with the data obtained in this study, strongly suggests the existence of a large northern Mediterranean olive fly population rather than several small and isolated populations. Gene flow and passive transport may be the reasons for the genetic similarity seen between the north Mediterranean populations. This information is of significant value in terms of the control of this pest.

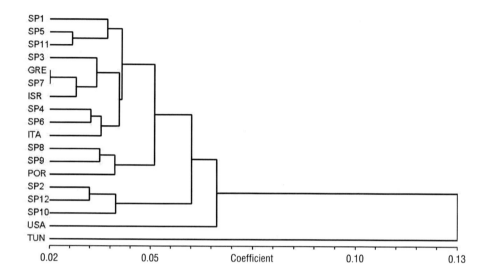

Figure 8. UPGMA dendrogram of *B. oleae* populations using Nei's genetic distances inferred from RAPD.

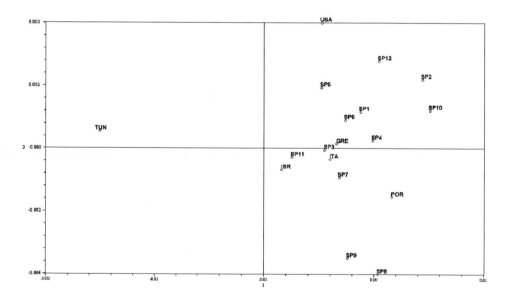

Figure 9 . Plot of the first two components in a principal component analysis of RAPD data from the eighteen populations of olive fruit fly sampled.

In addition, the American population tested, along with other sample from a previous study, showed a greater degree of within-population similarity than similarity with other populations, indicating it to be the product of a single introduction event and later dispersion.

In summary, phylogeographic studies involving RAPD markers have proven useful for characterizing the genetic structure of olive fly populations. A substantial level of polymorphism has been detected, along with considerable genetic diversity, though predominantly within populations (genetic diversity is low among populations). Strategies for future control programs should take this information into account. The low level of genetic differentiation among the north Mediterranean populations, and the important gene flow detected between them, show the need for integrated control programs coordinated between different geographical areas.

CONCLUSION

The classical methods of plant protection, i.e., the indiscriminate use and abuse of pesticides, have proven to be increasingly unsustainable and cost-ineffective due to the development of pest resistance, the rising financial costs of pesticide use, and the negative effects of pesticide use on human health and the environment (FAO, http://www.fao.org/).

Although the need to develop and implement more effective strategies of combating pests and pathogens has always been dire, the urgency of this challenge has increased sharply in recent years due to the globalisation of trade, the increase in the human population and therefore the increased demand for food, and social awakening with respect to health and biodiversity. Consumers have made clear that they want safer, more effective pest management methods while being able to protect the environment and their own health. The consensus is that better scientific knowledge of insect pests and their natural enemies could lead to more effective biological control. Certainly, molecular methodologies can provide us with new and useful information in this and other respects. Important questions related to population structure and dynamics can be answered through phylogeographic analysis using different molecular markers and technologies. This is important since the control of pests requires very different strategies depending on the variation present in and between different populations. A single bioinvasion and later expansion may need to be dealt with differently than several or continuing bioinvasions, as might a pest that has recently colonised an area compared to one that is long established. The same is true for large, widespread populations compared to a number of different populations, large populations compared to those that suffer periodic bottlenecks, and those with high gene flow compared to isolated populations, etc.

Scientific knowledge is the cornerstone on which to build success in Integrated Pest Management, and agricultural associations are now demanding the EU legislate on a scientific basis. Phylogeographic knowledge *must* be taken into account if we are to a fight insect pests, in a way that is more efficient, more cost-effective, and safer for our health and environment.

REFERENCES

Abrahamson, WG; Weis, AE (1997). *Evolutionary ecology across three trophic levels: Goldenrods, Gallmakers, and Natural Enemies.* Monographs in Population Biology 29, Princeton University Press.

Afonso, JM; Prestano J; Hernández, M. Rapid isolation of mitochondrial DNA from *Drosophila* adults. *Biochemical Genetics.* 26, 381-386. 1988.

Alberola, TM; Aptosoglou, S; Arsenakis, M; Bel, Y; Delrio, G; Ellar, DJ; Ferre, J; Granero, F; Guttmann, DM; Koliais, S; Martinez-Sebastian, MJ; Prota, R; Rubino, S; Satta, A; Scarpellini, G; Sivropoulou, A; Vasara, E. Insecticidal activity of strains of *Bacillus thuringiensis* on larvae and adults of *Bactrocera oleae* Gmelin (Diptera, Tephritidae). *Journal of Invertebrate Pathology* 74, 127-136. 1999.

Aluja, M; Mangan, RL. Fruit Fly (Diptera: Tephritidae) host status determination: critical conceptual, methodological, and regulatory considerations. *Annual Reviews of Entomology* 53, 473-502. 2008.

Augustinus, AA; Mamuris, Z; Stratikopoulos, EE; D'Amelio, S; Zacharopoulou, A; Mathiopoulos, KD. Microsatellite analysis of olive fly populations in the Mediterranean indicates a westward expansion of the species. *Genetica* 125, 231-241. 2005.

Avise, JC. Mitochondrial DNA and the evolutionary genetics of higher animals. *Philosophical Transactions of the Royal Society London B* 312:325-342. 1986.

Avise, JC. Matriarchal liberation. *Nature* 352:192. 1991.

Avise, JC. Ten unorthodox perspectives on evolution prompted by comparative population genetic findings on mitochondrial DNA. *Annual Review of Genetics* 25:45-69. 1991.

Avise, JC. (1994). *Molecular Markers, Natural History, and Evolution.* Chapman & Hall, New York (511 pp.).

Avise, JC. (2000). *Phylogeography: The History and Formation of Species.* Harvard University Press, Cambridge, MA. (447 pp.).

Avise, JC. An American naturalist's impressions on Australian biodiversity and conservation. *Biodiversity and Conservation* 12:1-7. 2003.

Avise, JC. The best and the worst of times for evolutionary biology. *BioScience* 53:247-255. 2003.

Avise, JC. 2004. *Molecular Markers, Natural History, and Evolution* (Second Edition). Sinauer, Sunderland, MA. (684 pp.).

Avise, JC; Arnold, J; Ball Jr., RM; Bermingham, E; Lamb, T; Neigel, J.E; Reeb, CA; Saunders, NC. Intraspecific phylogeography: the mitochondrial DNA bridge between population genetics and systematics. *Annual Review of Ecology and Systematics* 18:489-522. 1987.

Barranco, D; Fernández-Escobar, R; Rallo, L; Eds. (2004). *El cultivo del olivo.* Mundi-Prensa-Junta de Andalucia, España.

Baruffi, L; Damian, G; Guglielmino, CR; Bandi, C; Malacrida, AR; Gasperi, G. Polymorphism within and between populations of *Ceratitis capitata*: comparison between RAPD and multilocus enzyme electrophoresis data. *Heredity* 74, 425-437. 1995.

Behura, SK. Molecular marker systems in insects: current trends and future avenues. *Molecular ecology.* 15(11): 3087. 2006.

Beitia, F. Nueva especie de mosca blanca en las Islas Canarias. *Terralia*, 4: 24-25. 1998.

Bellows, TS; Fisher, TW eds.. (1999). *Handbook of Biological Control. Principles and applications of biological control*, Academic Press, New York, USA.

Bohonak, AJ; Davies, N; Villablanca, FX; Roderick, GK. Invasion genetics of New World medflies: testing alternative colonization scenarios. *Biological Invasions* 3: 103-111. 2001.

Bonizzoni, M; Malacrida, A.R; Guglielmino, CR; Gomulski, LM; Gasperi, G; Zheng, L. Microsatellite polymorphism in the Mediterranean fruit fly, *Ceratitis capitata. Insect Molecular Biology* 9, 251-261. 2000.

Bonizzoni, M; Zheng, L; Guglielmino, CR; Haymer, DS; Gasperi, G; Gomulski, LM; Malacrida, AR. Microsatellite analysis of medfly bioinfestations in California. *Molecular Ecology* 10:2515–2524. 2001.

Bonizzoni, M; Guglielmino, CR; Smallridge, CJ; Gomulski, LM; Malacrida, AR; Gasperi, G. On the origins of medfly invasion and expansion in Australia. *Molecular Ecology* 13: 3845-3855. 2004.

Bush, GL; Kitto, GB. Research on the genetic structure of wild and laboratory strains of the olive fly. FAO Report: *Development of pest management system for olive culture program.* Food and Agricultura Organization of the United Nations, Rome. 1979.

Callejas, C; Roda, P; Reyes, A; Ochando, MD. Identificación genética de *Dacus – Bactrocera- oleae* Gmelin (Diptera: Tephritidae) mediante marcadores RAPD-PCR. *Boletin de Sanidad Vegetal y Plagas* 24, 873-882. 1998.

Callejas, C; Ochando, MD. Allozymic variability in Spanish populations of *Ceratitis capitata. Fruits* 59, 181-190. 2004.

Callejas, C; Gobbi, A; Velasco, A; Beitia, FJ; Ochando, MD. The use of RAPD markers to detect genetic patterns in *Aleurodicus dispersus* (Hemiptera: Aleyrodidae) populations from the Canary Islands. *European Journal of Entomology*, 102, 289-291. 2005.

Carey, JR. Establishment of the Mediterranean fruit fly in California. *Science* 253, 1369-1373. 1991.

Coombs, J; Coombs, R. (2003). *A dictionary of Biological Control and Integrated Pest Management* (3rd Edition), 300 pp. CPL Press, Newbury, UK.

Cox, JSTH. (2007). The role of geographic information systems and spatial analysis in Area-Wide vector control programmes, pp.199-210, In *"Area-Wide control of Insect pests"*, Vreysen et al., eds., Springer, Dordrecht, The Netherlands.

Davies, N; Villablanca, FX; Roderick, GK. Bioinvasions of the Medfly *Ceratitis capitata*: source estimation using DNA sequences at multiple intron loci. *Genetics* 153: 351-360. 1999.

De Sousa, GB; de Dutari, GP; Gardenal, CN. Genetic structure of *Aedes albifasciatus* (Diptera: Culicidae) populations in Central Argentina determined by random amplified polymorphic DNA-polymerase chain reaction markers. *Journal of Medical Entomology* 36, 400-404. 1999.

Debach, P. (1964). *Biological control of insect pest and weeds*. Reinhold, New York, USA. 844 pp.

Dowell, RV; Krass, CJ. Exotic pests pose growing problem for California. *California Agriculture* 46: 6–12. 1992.

Downie, DA; Fisher, JR; Granett, J. Grapes, galls, and geography: the distribution of nuclear and mtDNA variation across host plant species and regions in a specialist herbivore. *Evolution* 55, 1345-1362. 2001.

European Environment Agency (EEA), Office for Official Publications of the European Communities (OPOCE). *Europe's environment — The fourth assessment.* European Environment Agency. Report No 1/2007. Copenhagen, Denmark.

Felsenstein, J. (2004). *Inferring Phylogenies.* Sinauer Associates, Sunderland, Massachusetts, USA.

Fimiani, P. (1989) Mediterranean region. pp. 37-55 *in* Robinson, A.S. & Hooper, G.H. (Eds.) *Fruit flies: Their Biology, Natural enemies and Control.* Vol. 3A. Elsevier, Amsterdam, The Netherlands.

Fletcher, B.S. (1989). Life history strategies of tephritid fruit flies. In *Fruit flies: their Biology, Natural Enemies and Control,* Vol 3A, eds. Robinson and Hooper: 195-208. Elsevier, Amsterdam.

Gallo, D.N.O., Wiendel, F.M., Silvera Neto, S. & Ricardo, P.L.C. (1970) *Manual de Entomologia Agronomica.* Ceres, Säo Paulo, Brasil.

Gasperi, G; Guglielmino, CR; Malacrida, AR; Milani, R. Genetic variability and gene flow in geographical populations of *Ceratitis capitata* (Wied.) (medfly). *Heredity* 67: 347-356. 1991.

Gasperi, G; Bonizzoni, M; Gomulski, LM; Murelli, V; Torti, C; Malacrida, AR;Guglielmino, CR. Genetic differentiation, gene flow and the origin of infestations of the medfly, *Ceratitis capitata. Genetica* 116: 125–135. 2002.

Gasparich, GE; Sheppard, WS; Han, HY; McPheron, BA; Steck, GJ. Analysis of mitochondrial DNA and development of PCR-based diagnostic molecular markers for the Mediterranean fruit fly (*Ceratitis capitata*) populations. *Insect Molecular Biology* 4, 61-67. 1995.

Gasparich, GE; Silva, JG; Han, HY; McPheron, BA; Steck, GJ; Sheppard, WS. Population genetic structure of Mediterranean Fruit Fly (Diptera: Tephritidae) and Implications for Worldwide Colonization Patterns. *Annals of the Entomological Society of America* 90: 790-797. 1997.

Gomulski, LM; Bourtzis, K; Brogna, S; Morandi, PA; Bonvicini, C; Sebastiani, F; Torit, C; Guglielmino, CR; Savakis, C; Gasperi, G; Malacrida, AR. Intron size polymorphism of the *Adh1* gene parallels the worldwide colonization history of the Mediterranean fruit fly, *Ceratitis capitata. Molecular Ecology* 7: 1729-1741. 1998.

Greathead, DJ; Greathead AH. Biological control of insect pests by insect parasitoids and predators: the BIOCAT database. *Biocontrol News Information* 13: 61N–68N. 1992.

Hagen, KS; William, WW; Tassan, RL. Mediterranean fruit fly: The worst may be yet to come. *California Agriculture* (University of California, Division of Agricultural Sciences, Reports of progress in research), March-April 1981, 35: 5–7. 1981.

Haymer, S; McInnis, DO. Resolution of populations of the Mediterranean fruit fly at the DNA level using random primers for the polymerase chain reaction. *Genome* **37**: 244-248. 1994.

He, M; Haymer, S. Genetic relationships of populations and the origins of new infestations of the Mediterranean fruit fly. *Molecular Ecology* 8, 1247-1257. 1999.

Headrick, DH; Goeden, RD. Issues concerning the eradication or establishment and biological control of the Mediterranean fruit fly, *Ceratitis capitata* (Wiedemann) (Diptera: Tephritidae) in California. *Biological Control* **6**, 412-421. 1996.

Heckel, DG. Genomics in pure and applied entomology. *Annual Review of Entomology* 48, 235-260. 2003.

Hernández-Suárez, E; Carnero, A; Hernández, M; Beitia, F; Alonso, C. *Lecanoideus floccissimus* (Homoptera, Aleyrodidae): Nueva plaga en las Islas Canarias. *Phytoma-ESPAÑA* 91: 35-48. 1997.

Hernández-Suárez E. (1999). *La familia Aleyrodidae y sus enemigos naturales en las Islas Canarias*. PhD Thesis, Universidad de La Laguna (Tenerife, Islas Canarias), 687pp.

Higuchi, R., 1989, Simple and rapid preparation of samples for PCR, in H.A. Erlich (ed) *PCR Technology* (New York: Stockton Press), pp: 31-38.

Hillis, DM; Moritz, C; Mable, BK. (1996) *Molecular Systematics*. 2 edition. Sinauer Associates Inc., Sunderland, MA, USA.

Huettel, MD; Fuerst, PA; Maruyama, M; Chakraborty, R. Genetic effects of multiple population bottlenecks in the Mediterranean fruit fly (*Ceratitis capitata*). *Genetics* 94s, 47 (abstract). 1980.

Kourti, A. Comparison of mtDNA variants among Mediterranean and New World introductions of the Mediterranean fruit fly *Ceratitis capitata* (Wied.). *Biochemical Genetics* **35**, 363-370. 1997.

Kourti, A. Patterns of variation within and between Greek populations of *Ceratitis capitata* suggest extensive gene flow and latitudinal clines. *Journal of Economic Entomology* 93, 1186-1190. 2004.

Lin, H; Downie, DA; Walker, MA; Granett, J; English-Loeb, G. Genetic structure in native populations of grape phylloxera (Homoptera: Phylloxeridae). *Annals of the Entomological Society of America* 92, 376-381. 1999.

Lomolino, MV; Riddle, BR; Brown, JH. (2006). *Biogeography*. Sinauer Assocciates, Inc. Sunderland, Massachusetts, USA.

Loukas, M. (1989) Population genetic studies of fruit flies of economic importance, specially medfly and olive fruit fly, using electrophoretic methods. pp. 69-102 *in* Loxdale, H.J. & den Hollander, J. (Eds.) *Electrophoretic Studies on Agricultural Pests*. Clarendon Press, Oxford, United Kingdom.

Loxdale, HD; Lushai, G. Molecular markers in entomology (Review). *Bulletin of Entomological Research* 88, 577 – 600. 1998.

Malacrida, AR; Guglielmino, CR; Gasperi, G; Baruffi, L; Milani, R. Spatial and temporal differentiation in colonizing populations of *Ceratitis capitata*. *Heredity* 69, 101-111. 1992.

Malacrida, AR; Marinoni, F; Tori, C; Gomulski, LM; Sebastián, F; Bonvicini, C; Gasperi, G; Guglielmino, CR. Genetic aspects of the worldwide colonization process of *Ceratitis capitata*. *The Journal of Heredity* 89, 501-507. 1998.

Malacrida, AR; Gomulski, LM; Bonizzoni, M; Bertin, S; Gasperi, G; Guglielmino, CR. Globalization and fruit fly invasion and expansion: the medfly paradigm. *Genetica* 131: 1–9. 2007.

Martin, JH; Mifsud, D; Rapisarda, C. The whiteflies (Hemiptera:Aleyrodidae) of Europe and the Mediterranean Basin. *Bulletin of Entomological Reserach* 90: 407-448. 2000.

Mayurama, T. Effective number of alleles in a subdivided population. *Theoretical Population Biology* 1, 273-306. 1970.

Mayurama T. Distribution of gene frequencies in a geographically structured finite population. I. Distribution of neutral genes and of genes with a small effect. *Annals of Human Genetics* 35, 411-423. 1972.

Mcpheron, BA; Gasparich, GE; Han, H-Y; Steck, GJ; Sheppard, WS. Mitochondrial DNA restriction map for the Mediterranean fruit fly, *Ceratitis capitata. Biochemical Genetics* 32: 25-33. 1994.

Meixner, MD; McPheron, BA; Silva, JG; Gasparich, GE; Sheppard, WS. The Mediterranean fruit fly in California: evidence for multiple introductions and persistent populations based on microsatellite and mitochondrial DNA variability. *Molecular Ecology* 11: 891–899. 2002.

Mendelson, TC; Shaw, KL. Use of AFLP markers in surveys of arthropod diversity. *Methods in Enzymology*, 395: 161-177. 2005.

Nardi, F; Carapelli, A; Dallai, R; Roderick, GK; Frati, F. Population structure and colonization history of the olive fly, *Bactrocera oleae* (Diptera, Tephritidae). *Molecular Ecology* 14, 2729-2738. 2005.

Nei, M; Li, WH. Mathematical model for studying genetic variation in terms of restriction endonucleases. *Proceedings of the National Academy of Sciences. USA* 76, 5269-5273. 1979.

Nei, M; Tajima, F. DNA polymorphism detectable by restriction endonucleases. *Genetics* 97, 145-163. 1981.

Nei, M; Kumar, S. (2000) *Molecular Evolution and Phylogenetics.* Oxford University Press, New York, USA.

Ochando, MD; Callejas, C; Fernández, OH; Reyes, A. Variabilidad genética aloenzimática en *Dacus oleae* (Gmelin) (Díptera: Tephritidae) I. Análisis de dos poblaciones naturales del sureste español. *Boletín de Sanidad Vegetal y Plagas*, 20, 35-44. 1994.

Ochando, MD; Reyes, A. Genetic population structure in olive fly *Bactrocera oleae* (Gmelin): gene flow and patterns of geographic differentiation. *Journal of Applied Entomology* 124, 177-183. 2000.

Ochando, MD; Reyes, A.; Callejas, C; Segura, D and Fernández, P. Molecular genetic methodologies applied to the study of fly pests. *Trends in Entomology,* 3, 73-85. 2003a.

Ochando, MD; Reyes, A; Callejas, C. Genetic structure of *Ceratitis capitata* species: within and between population variability. *Integrated Control in Citrus Fruit Crops. IOBC/wprs Bulletin* 26 (6): 59-72. 2003b.

Ochando, MD; Beroiz, B; Callejas, C; Hernández-Crespo, P; Ortego, F; Castañera, C. Genética poblacional de *Ceratitis capitata* mediante el empleo de marcadores moleculares. *Levante Agrícola*, 385, 139-144. 2007.

Reyes, A. (1995) Análisis de la variabilidad genética en poblaciones españolas de *Ceratitis capitata* Wied. mediante la utilización de marcadores moleculares. Ph. D. Thesis. Complutense University, Madrid, Spain, pp. 202.

Reyes, A; Ochando, MD. A study of gene-enzyme variability in three Spanish populations of Ceratitis capitata. *International Organization for Biological Control. West Palaeartic Regional Section Bulletin* 17, 151-160. 1994.

Reyes, A; Linacero, R; Ochando, MD. Molecular genetics and integrated control: A universal genomic DNA microextraction mehtod for PCR, RAPD, restriction and Southern análisis. *IOBC/wprs Bulletin* 20 (4): 274-284. 1997.

Reyes, A; Ochando, MD. Genetic differentiation in Spanish populations of *Ceratitis capitata* as revealed by abundant soluble proteins. *Genetica* 104, 59-66. 1998a.

Reyes, A; Ochando, MD. Use of molecular markers for detecting the geographical origin of *Ceratitis capitata* (Diptera:Tephritidae) populations. *Annals of the Entomological Society of America* 91, 222-227. 1998b.

Reyes, A; Ochando, MD. Mitochondrial DNA variation in Spanish populations of *Ceratitis capitata* (Wiedeman) (Tephrtidae) and the colonization process. *Journal of Applied Entomology* 128, 358-364. 2004.

Rice, RE. Bionomics of the olive fruit fly *Bactrocera (Dacus) oleae*. Plant Protection Quaterly 10, 1-5. 2000.

Rice, RE; Phillips, PA; Stewart-Leslie, J; Sibbett, GS. Olive fruit fly populations measured in central and southern California. *California Agriculture* 57, 122-127. 2003.

Robinson, AS; Hooper, G. (1989). *Fruit flies, their biology, natural enemies and control.* Elsevier Amsterdam, The Netherlands.

Roderick, GK; Navajas, M. Genotypes in novel environments: Genetics and evolution in biological control. *Nature Reviews Genetics* 4, 889-899. 2003.

Ruiz, A. (1948). *Fauna entomológica del olivo en España. Estudio sistemático y biológico de las especies de mayor importancia económica.* Trabajos del Instituto Español de Entomología. Madrid, Spain.

Segura, D; Callejas, C; Ochando, MD. Molecular markers as useful tools for population genetics of the olive fly, *Bactrocera oleae. IOBC wprs Bulletin,* 30, 79-87. 2007.

Segura, D; Callejas, C; Ochando, MD. *Bactrocera oleae*: a single large population in the Northern Mediterranean basin. *Journal of Applied Entomology,* 132, 706-713. 2008.

Severson, SE; Brown, B; Knudson, DL. Genetic and physical mapping in mosquitoes: molecular approaches. *Annual Review of Entomology* 46, pp. 183–219. 2001.

Sheppard, WS; Steck, GJ; McPheron, BA. Geographic populations of the medfly may be differentiated by mitochondrial DNA variation. *Experientia* 48, 1010-1013. 1992.

Silva, J; Mexner, M; McPheron, B; Steck, G; Sheppard, W. Recent Mediterranean fruit fly (Diptera: Tephritidae) infestations in Florida. A genetic perspective. *Journal of Economic Entomology* 96, 1711–1718. 2003.

Steck, GJ; Gasparich, GE; Han, HY; McPheron, BA; Sheppard, WS. Distribution of mitochondrial DNA haplotypes among *Ceratitis capitata* populations worldwide. pp. 291-296 *in* McPheron, B.A. & Steck, G.J. (Eds.) *Fruit fly pests. A world assessment of their biology and management.* St. Lucie Press, Delray Beach, FL, USA. 1996

Swofford, DL; Olsen, GJ; Waddell, PJ; Hillis, DM. (1996). Phylogenetic inference pp. 407-514, in *Molecular Systematics*, Hillis, D.M., Moritz, C., Mable, B.K. eds., Sinauer Assoc., Sunderland, MA, USA.

Tan, K-H ed. (2000). *Area-wide control of fruit flies and other insect pests*. IAEA. *Sinaran Bros. Sdn. Bhd* Penerbit University Sains Malasia, 782 pp.

Unruh, TR; Woolley, JB. (1999). Molecular methods in classical biological methods. In *"Handbook of Biological Control"*, Bellows and Fisher, eds., Academic Press, New York, USA.

Villablanca, FX; Roderick, GK; Palumbi, SR. Invasion genetics of the Mediterranean fruit fly: variation in multiple nuclear introns. *Molecular Ecology* 7: 547–560. 1998.

Vreysen, MJ B; Robinson, AS; Hendrichs, J. (Eds.) 2007. *Area-wide Control of Insect Pests: From Research to Field Implementation.* Springer, Dordrecht, The Netherlands. 789 pp.

Waterhouse, DF; Norris, KR. (1989). *Aleurodicus dispersus* spiraling whitefly. pp. 12-23. In: Biological Control Pacific Prospects - Supplement 1. Australian Center for International Agriculture Research, Canberra, Australia.

Welsh, J; McClelland, M. Fingerprinting genomes using PCR with arbitrary primers. *Nucleic Acids Research* 18, 7213-7218. 1990.

Williams, JKG; Kubelik, AR; Livak, KJ; Rafalsky, JA; Tyngey, SV. DNA polymorphisms amplified by arbitrary primers are useful as genetic markers. *Nucleic Acids Research* 18, 6531-6535. 1990.

Wright, S. Evolution in Mendelian populations. *Genetics* 16, 97-159. 1931.

Yong. HS. Allozyme variation in the melon fly *Dacus cucurbitae* (Insecta: Diptera: Tephritidae) from Peninsular Malaysia. *Comparative Biochemistry and Physiology* 102B, 367-370. 1992.

Zhang, DX; Hewitt, GM. Insect mitochondrial control region: a review of its structure, evolution and usefulness in evolutionary studies. *Biochemical Systematics and Ecology* 25: 99-120. 1997.

Zitoudi, K; Margaritopoulos, JT; Mamuris, Z; Tsitsipis, JA. Genetic variation in *Myzus persicae* populations associated with host-plant and life cycle category. *Entomologia Experimentalis et Applicata* 99, 303-311. 2001.

Zouros, E; Loukas, M. (1989). Biochemical and colonization genetics of *Dacus oleae* (Gmelin). In: *Fruit flies, Their biology, Natural enemies and Control.* A. S. Robinson and G. Hooper (eds.). Chapter 5.3, 75-87.

In: Phylogeography
Editor: Damien S. Rutgers

ISBN: 978-1-60692-954-4
© 2013 Nova Science Publishers, Inc.

Chapter 3

HOST SPECIFICITY AND SPECIATION IN PARASITIC PLANTS

Chris J. Thorogood and Simon J. Hiscock
University of Bristol, Bristol, UK

ABSTRACT

Parasitic plants have aroused curiosity among scientists for centuries, yet they remain one of the most poorly understood groups of flowering plants (angiosperms), and much of their evolutionary biology remains a mystery. There are approximately 4,000 species of parasitic plants (in 19 families) which occur in all major biomes, from arctic islands to tropical forests. The evolutionary shift to parasitism has been associated with the degeneration of morphological features traditionally used in plant classification to infer evolutionary relationships, making systematic studies of the relationships between parasitic plants and their photosynthetic ancestors extremely difficult. Therefore until very recently, our understanding of the evolutionary origins of parasitic angiosperms has lagged behind that of other major groups of angiosperms.

Parasitic plants show considerable variation in their host specificity. For example, some species infect hundreds of species from taxonomically diverse families, while others are restricted to a single host species. Host ecology may isolate parasite populations and facilitate genetic divergence. For example in leaf-eating (phytophagus) insects which, like parasitic plants, are discriminate users with respect to the host plants on which they feed, host specificity has been demonstrated to drive genetic divergence, and ultimately speciation. However speciation in parasitic plants has, until recently, remained relatively unexplored by evolutionary biologists, and our understanding of host specificity as a potential catalyst for speciation in these plants has lagged behind that of phytophagus insects. Now, in light of recent research, a similar pattern of host-driven speciation in parasitic plants is emerging. This chapter reviews recent research into the host specificity of parasitic plants, which appears to be an important and underestimated promoter of genetic divergence and speciation.

PARASITIC PLANTS

Parasitic plants attach to the roots and shoots of autotrophic plants from which they extract water, nutrients and organic solutes via a haustorium – a multicellular intrusive organ that penetrates host tissues to absorb nutrients. It has been estimated that about 1% of flowering plants are parasitic (Kuijt, 1969), and these plants are found in all major biomes, from arctic islands to tropical forests (Press and Phoenix, 2005). They have been described as keystone species and ecosystem engineers, because they generate profound effects on plant community structure (Press and Graves 1995; Press and Phoenix 2005), yet surprisingly they have been largely ignored in community theory, and our understanding of parasitic angiosperms and their interactions with their host plants lags behind that of other plant-pathogen and symbiotic associations in plants (Press and Graves 1995). Parasitic plants are a taxonomically diverse group of angiosperms that can be broadly categorised as either root- or stem- parasites according to the point of attachment to their host plants (Musselman and Press, 1995; Heide-Jørgenson, 2008). The degree of dependence on host-derived nutrition has also been used to categorise parasitic plants into two groups: (i) hemiparasites, which have retained photosynthesis and (ii) holoparasites, which derive all photosynthates from their hosts (Randle and Wolfe, 2005). Many holoparasites show extreme reductions in morphology, lacking leaves, stems and roots (Young et al., 1999), and some are barely recognisable as plants at all. Following the evolutionary transition from autotrophy to heterotrophy, this extreme divergence from their ancestral photosynthetic species has impeded the resolution of phylogenetic affinities in holoparasitic plants (Young et al., 1999; Nickrent et al., 2004; Davis et al., 2007). However, recent advances in molecular phylogenetics are now revealing the first objective insights into the evolutionary origins of this enigmatic group of plants.

Most research into parasitic plants has been directed at the obstacle to agriculture these plants represent where they parasitize commercial crops (Parker and Riches, 1993). However studies have also demonstrated that parasitic plants offer a platform for exploring plastid genome evolution in the absence of the plastid's primary function, photosynthesis (dePamphilis, 1995; Bungard, 2004). Plastid genomes in nonphotosynthetic holoparasitic plants have undergone extreme reductions in gene content (dePamphilis et al., 1997). However portions of the genome necessary for functions unrelated to photosynthesis have been retained, so the plastid genome in these plants represents an ideal model with which to investigate plastid gene function (dePamphilis and Palmer, 1990; Wimpee et al., 1991; dePamphilis, 1995; dePamphilis et al., 1997; Wolfe and dePamphilis, 1998; Bungard, 2004). More recently, parasitic plants have also presented the opportunity to investigate horizontal gene transfer (the exchange of genes across mating barriers: HGT) in flowering plants. For example, Davis and Wurdack (2004) demonstrated that part of the mitochondrial genome in the gigantic holoparasite *Rafflesia* was acquired from host plant species via an HGT-event. The full extent of HGT between parasitic angiosperms and their hosts has not been ascertained, and present-day hosts may not be the only conduit for host-parasite gene transfer if host latitude has shifted through time during the evolution of parasite lineages (Nickrent et al., 2004). Taken together, these studies demonstrate that parasitic angiopserms provide a unique opportunity for studying genome evolution in plants. A series of recent studies suggest that parasitic plants may also be ideal models for investigating host-driven patterns of speciation. This chapter reviews research into host specificity from the cellular to the ecosystem level in parasitic plants, and then explores how this process can act as a template for population divergence, and ultimately, speciation. An emerging trend suggests that host specificity is a significant evolutionary driving force in parasitic plants, therefore these organisms offer a unique platform for investigating patterns of host-associated speciation.

THE SEARCH FOR PHOTOSYNTHETIC ANCESTORS

Identifying the free-living relatives of parasitic organisms presents a phylogenetic dilemma - particularly in the case of parasitic flowering angiosperms, in which the evolutionary origins remain largely unclear (Barkman et al., 2007). Root grafting has been speculated to have preceded parasitism in root parasites, whereas in stem parasites, a twining habit is likely to have been an important precursor to parasitism (Kuijt, 1969). A molecular hypothesis for evolution and genome reduction in parasitic plants was first proposed by Searcy (1970). This hypothesis stated that a free-living ancestor developed a symbiotic relationship with its host plant, following which selection pressures on features associated with the free-living form were relaxed. This transition was followed by the loss of biochemical pathways, (the products of which were provided by the host), and a reduction in morphological features, that culminated in obligate parasitism. The genes that originally encoded these reduced features then accumulated random mutations under relaxed selection pressures, and were eventually deleted from the genome (Searcy 1970; Searcy and MacInnis, 1970; dePamphilis, 1995). Indeed, extant holoparasites show extreme reductions in gross morphological features and plastid genome size, and this divergence from their photosynthetic ancestors, has hindered the resolution of phylogenetic affinities in parasitic angiosperms (Young et al., 1999; Nickrent et al., 2004; Davis et al., 2007); of the 18 families listed as "position uncertain" in a recent molecular-based Angiosperm Phylogeny Group (APG) classification of flowering plants, seven were families of holoparasites (APG, 2003). However recent advances in molecular phylogenetics, coupled with broader sampling strategies, have begun to elucidate the evolutionary origins of parasitic plants.

A recent phylogenetic analysis of 102 species of seed plants using three mitochondrial genes revealed at least 11 independent origins of parasitism in the angiosperms, eight of which consisted entirely of holoparasitic species (Barkman et al., 2007). This study also suggested that the diversity of modern-day parasites has evolved disproportionately from particular lineages, for example the monocots, campanulids and caryophyllids (22%, 12% and 7% of angiosperm diversity respectively), have no parasitic representatives. In contrast the lamiids alone (23% of angiosperm diversity) have independently evolved parasitism three times. The parasitic angiosperms are clearly a taxonomically diverse group of plants (Figure 1), united only by their mode of nutrition, but why particular angiosperm lineages may have had an evolutionary predisposition to parasitism remains a mystery.

The phylogenetic positioning of some families of parasitic angiosperms has been particularly challenging, and their relationships have remained elusive until very recently. For example, the poorly understood Hydnoraceae (Figure 2), has been the source of much disagreement among taxonomists in the past.

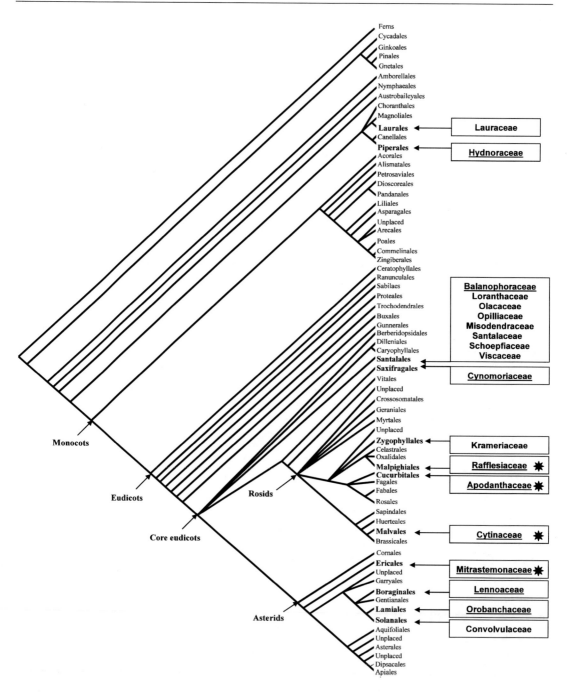

Figure 1. The phylogenetic distribution of orders among the angiosperms that have evolved parasitism (indicated in bold). This tree gives an approximate estimation of the taxonomic breadth of parasitic plant evolution which has evolved at 11-13 times and occurs in 19 families (Barkman et al., 2007). Underlined families are holoparasitic, and families with stars are endophytic. Tree based on data from the Angiosperm Phylogeny Group.

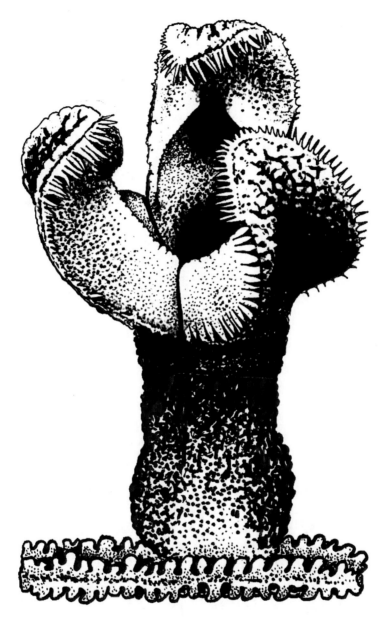

Nickrent et al., 2002

Figure 2. The curious flower of *Hydnora africana* (Hydnoraceae) emerged from a pilot root attached to the host root (shrubs in the Euphorbiaceae in southern Africa). The flower emits the strong smell of carrion to attract insects which become trapped to ensure pollination. Molecular data have now placed the previously phylogenetically elusive Hydnoraceae with the basal Aristolochiaceae.

The highly modified vegetative and floral features of this family of holoparasites rendered reliable classifications based on morphology impossible (Nickrent et al., 2002). Traditionally, this family was erroneously allied with the Rafflesiales (Cronquist, 1988; Takhtajan, 1997), probably on account of the convergence of flesh-coloured carrion flowers. However the combined use of nuclear, mitochondrial and chloroplast DNA sequence data revealed association between the Hydnoraceae and the Aristolochiaceae (Nickrent et al., 2002) – a basal group of angiosperms in the Piperales. The hydnoraceae consists of two genera: *Hydnora* in tropical Africa and Madagascar, and *Prosopanche* in South America. These root parasites produce thick, cable-like roots from which the extraordinary flowers emerge above ground and emit the smell of carrion to attract pollinating flies and beetles (Molau, 1995). Species in the Hydnoraceae are often highly host-specific, therefore divergence on host plants with distinct ecological niches may have been the driver of speciation in these plants.

Another poorly understood order of holoparasitic plants was previously classified as the Balanophorales, - a grossly reduced, fungus-like group of plants that consisted of two families, the Balanophoraceae (Figure 3A) and the Cynomoriaceae (Figure 3B). The monogeneric Cynomoriaceae has long been known in Chinese medicine, however the photosynthetic relatives of these plants remained elusive until recently. Nickrent et al., (2005) reported a molecular phylogenetic analysis of nuclear ribosomal DNA and mitochondrial *matR* sequence data, that strongly supported the independent origin of the Balanophoraceae and the Cynomoriaceae. In this analysis, the Balanophoraceae was placed near the Santalales – a largely tropical and subtropical order that includes many hemiparasites such as mistletoes, while the Cynomoriaceae is derived from the Saxifragales - a morphologically diverse group that includes annual and perennial herbs, succulents, shrubs, vines, and trees. This analysis refuted all previous classifications that grouped the Balanophoraceae with the Cynomoriaceae on account of their convergent morphological features, such as fungus-like inflorescences that bear numerous, densely packed tiny flowers.

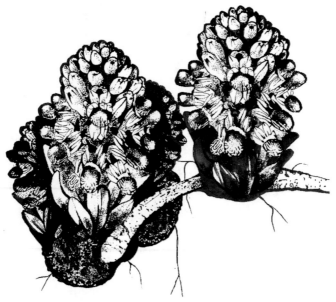

Nickrent et al., 2005.

Figure 3 A. Inflorescences of *Balanophora fungosa* (Balanophoraceae) attached to a host root; B. The Inflorescence of *Cynomorium coccineum* (Cynomoriaceae) characterised by its densely packed, highly reduced flowers. Previous classifications based on morphology indicated these families were of monophyletic origin; molecular data have now placed the Balanophoraceae with the Santalales, and the Cynomoriaceae with the Saxafragales respectively.

The most taxonomically challenging of all parasitic plants are the highly specialised endophytic holoparasites (Figure 4), which live within the tissues of their hosts for at least part of their life cycle, and have evolved independently in at least four lineages: Cytinaceae, Mitrostemonaceae, Apodanthaceae and Rafflesiaceae (Nickrent et al., 2004; Barkman et al., 2007). Many families of endophytic holoparasites of uncertain phylogenetic placement were traditionally 'lumped' in the Rafflesiales in the broadest sense, implying a monophyletic origin of these lineages (Davis, 2008). In contrast with these traditional classifications based on morphology, a multigene phylogenetic analysis recently supported the independent origin of these lineages. For example, the Cytinaceae (Figure 4A) – a family of holoparasites traditionally ascribed to the Rafflesiales on account of their endophytic growth habit (Nickrent et al., 2004) has now been identified to be sister to the Muntingiaceae (Malvales) – a small American family of woody plants, in a molecular phylogenetic analysis based on nuclear small-subunit rDNA and three chloroplast genes (Nickrent, 2007). All *Cytinus* species show reductions in gross morphological features, with vestigial scale-like leaves and the complete absence of functional external roots. The vegetative body of *Cytinus* is reduced to an endophytic system that ramifies within the tissues of the host plant, and is comparable with a fungal mycelium, therefore to all intents and purposes, the plant is only visible when in flower (deVega et al., 2008). Similarly problematic, the monogeneric Mitrostemonaceae (Figure 4B) comprises two widely disjunct species in both the Old and New World, that are parasitic on trees in the Fagaceae. This family has now been placed in the Ericales (Nickrent et al., 2004) – a relationship not previously proposed by taxonomists. The taxonomic perplexity associated with these families exemplifies the challenge faced by botanists that highly reduced endophytic holoparasites represent, and the confusion that has been associated with their classification based on morphological features in the past.

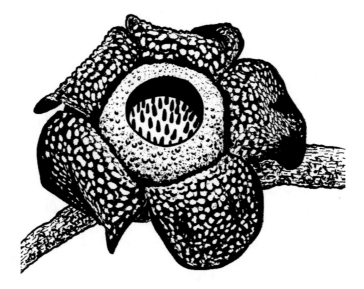

Figure 4. Endophytic parasites that were previously considered to be of monophyletic origin, and placed in the Rafflesiales, now identified to comprise four distinct linieages: A. *Cytinus hypocistis* (Cytinaceae) on host *Cistus* sp. root; B. *Mitrastema matudae* (Mitrastemonaceae) on host root; C. *Rafflesia arnoldii* (Rafflesiaceae) on host *Tetrastigma* sp. root; D. *Pilostyles thurberi* (Apodanthaceae) on host tree branch.

The enigmatic *Rafflesia* spp. *sensu stricto* (Rafflesiaceae) famously produce the largest flowers on earth, measuring up to one metre in diameter and weighing up tp 7 kg (Davis et al., 2007). The extreme reductions in morphological features of *Rafflesia* spp have deprived taxonomists of characters with which to infer their evolutionary origins. *Rafflesia* is a leafless, rootless non-photosynthetic parasite (Figure 4C), which lives endophytically as a mycelium-like mass within the tissues of its host plants (dePamphilis et al., 1997) - tropical vines in the Vitaceae. Elucidating the evolutionary origins of *Rafflesia* has been notoriously problematic until very recently (Davis, 2008). The first molecular phylogenetic studies placed the Rafflesiaceae in the Malpighiales, one of the most diverse angiosperm lineages (Barkman et al., 2004). Then, by sequencing multiple gene regions in species from a diverse cross-section of the Malpighiales, the Rafflesiaceae was finally resolved and embedded in the Euphorbiaceae, a surprising affinity given that this family is characterised by minute flowers which measure just a few millimetres across (Davis et al., 2007). A combination of detailed phylogenetic information and data on flower size estimated that the stem lineage of the Rafflesiaceae diverged from their minute-flowered ancestors at an incredible 91 times faster than the rest of the phylogeny (Davis et al., 2007). In spite of the notoriety of *Rafflesia*, surprisingly little is known about the evolutionary divergence or speciation of these extraordinary plants (Davis, 2008), and the genus has received inadequate systematic attention. Each of the 17 recognised species of *Rafflesia* are specific to just one or two of the 95 species of *Tetrastigma* vine (Vitaceae) that have been recorded in tropical Southeast Asia (Nais, 2001). Isolation of *Rafflesia* populations on host vines with differing ecologies and distributions, followed by genetic divergence, may have driven speciation in this genus, yet speciation in the Rafflesiaceae, as in many families of parasitic plants, remains unexplored.

Finally, the positioning of the last remaining lineage of endophytic holoparasites - the tiny-flowered Apodanthaceae, remains unsolved; mitochondrial *matR* and nuclear SSU rDNA data indicate either a relationship with Malvales or Cucurbitales (Nickrent ct al., 2004), but the closest photosynthetic relatives of this family of stem-parasites remain a mystery.

KEYSTONE SPECIES AND ECOSYSTEM ENGINEERS

Few studies have investigated the impacts of parasitic plants in their natural plant communities, and they have been largely ignored in plant community theory (Press and Graves, 1995; Press and Phoenix, 2005). However from the studies that have been conducted, an emerging consensus suggests that parasitic plants generate profound ecological impacts on plant communities in which they occur. Parasitism has major impacts on host growth, allometry and reproduction, which has the potential to drive shifts in the competitive balance between host and non-host species, and therefore plant community structure (Press and Phoenix, 2005; Phoenix and Press, 2005). Thus parasitic plants have been described as keystone species. In addition, on account of key traits such as dual autotrophic and heterotrophic carbon assimilation coupled with nutrient concentration, parasitic plants can significantly alter their surrounding environment, and are also considered to be 'ecosystem engineers' (Press and Phoenix, 2005). These ecological impacts may be far-reaching since parasitic plants occur in natural and semi-natural ecosystems from tropical rainforests to the high Arctic (Press, 1998), and account for *c.* 1% of all flowering plants (Kuijt, 1969).

The impacts parasitic plants have on natural plant communities are a direct consequence of their host specificity (Press and Phoenix, 2005). Host latitude in many parasitic plants is broad, however the number of 'preferred' hosts (i.e. on which parasites show optimal fitness) is often more restricted (Press and Graves 1995). Therefore while there may be many potential hosts in the plant community, those parasitized represent a subset of those available (Press and Phoenix, 2005). Parasitic plants can significantly influence the fitness of the host plants to which they are attached (Cameron et al., 2005). However, the effects on different species of host can also be disproportionate; for example *Rhinanthus minor* (Orobanchaceae, ex-Scrophulariaceae) shows a choice-for-choice host preference for grasses. In natural communities, this has been established to reduce grass biomass, and facilitate an increase in forb (broad-leaved plants other than grasses) diversity and abundance (Davies et al., 1997). Although *R. minor* extracts a significant biomass from host grasses, little repression of growth is observed in parasitized forbs (Cameron et al., 2008). It appears that forbs remain undamaged in contrast with grasses and leguminous hosts as a result of the defence response to haustorial invasion observed in the roots of these hosts (Cameron et al., 2006). Therefore differential parasite success, coupled with detrimental effects on host fitness, may underpin shifts in the relative species composition of plant communities in which parasitic plants occur (Cameron et al., 2005; Press and Phoenix, 2005). Conversely, where preferred hosts are competitively subordinate, parasitism can reduce species diversity by facilitating the greater dominance of the most abundant species (Gibson and Watkinson, 1989).

Rhinanthus minor has become a useful model for studying community-level interactions between host and parasite, on account of its broad host range which facilitates a spectrum of potential host responses to be examined (Gibson and Watkinson, 1989; Cameron et al., 2005; Cameron et al., 2006; Cameron et al., 2008). The ecological effects and plant community dynamics of other species of parasitic plant remain relatively unexplored, but the studies carried out to date indicate similar keystone effects. For example an experiment in which the hemiparasite *Triphysaria* (Scrophulariaceae) was artificially removed from a coastal prairie community in California, USA suggested the presence of this species in mixed stands of hosts facilitated the release of eudicot species from competition with grasses (Marvier, 1998) Similarly, holoparasitic dodders (*Cuscuta,* Convolvulariaceae) may also exert community level effects in the ecosystems in which they occur; Callaway and Pennings (1998) found that *C. salina* showed a strong host species preference for *Salicornia virginica*, the dominant competitor of saltmarshes in California, USA. In plots infected with *Cuscuta* over a three year period, *Salicornia* decreased in abundance, and the cover of another species, *Arthrocnemum,* increased by 558 % in just one year relative to the uninfected plots. Therefore by weakening the competitive dominant, *Cuscuta* enhanced community structure and diversity. Frequently the most heavily parasitized species are competitively dominant species, and parasitism facilitates the maintenance of competitively subordinate species (Press, 1998). No other studies to date have studied the effects of holoparasites on plant community structure which may be a consequence of their experimental intractability. Holoparasites can extract significant resources from their hosts (e.g. 20 % of host resources in *Orobanche*, Hibberd et al., 1999), and could potentially drive shifts in plant community structure by suppressing host species fitness discriminately, since these plants are often highly host-specific (Molau, 1995). Therefore it is not unreasonable to expect that as keystone species they may be as effective as hemiparasites, if not more so.

Parasitic plants have also been described as ecosystem engineers (Press and Phoenix, 2005), in that they modulate resource availability by changing the physical state of biotic and abiotic materials (Jones et al., 1994). For example, root hemiparasites alter their local environment by transforming materials from one physical state to another, which can have important consequences on nutrient cycling in nutrient-poor communities (Press and Phoenix, 2005). Parasitic plants generally have higher concentrations of foliar nutrients (such as phosphorous, magnesium and nitrogen) than their hosts (Pate, 1995), therefore hemiparasites that concentrate nutrients in their leaves have the potential to produce leaf litter that releases nutrients otherwise locked in host tissues, or in slowly decomposing plant litter (Quested et al., 2001; Quested, 2008). For example, in a study that compared the N, P and C content of leaf litter in seven species of root hemiparasitic Scrophulariaceae with nine species of commonly co-occurring dwarf shrubs, graminoids and herbs, the litter from the hemiparasites contained between 1.8 and 8.5 times more N as the litter of the commonly co-occurring non-parasites (Quested et al., 2001). Thus, in the nutrient-limited environments in which these hemiparasites tend to occur, they may have significant impacts on plant community structure, suggesting that parasitic plants must be considered integral components in plant community and ecosystem theory (Press and Phoenix, 2005; Quested, 2008).

HOST SPECIFICITY

Host specificity in parasitic plants is determined by the compatibility of host-parasite interactions at the biochemical and molecular level, as well as by host distribution and parasite dispersal potential at the population level (Heide-Jørgenson, 2008). Most parasitic plants can potentially parasitize a diverse range of hosts, and are thus considered to be generalists (Kelly et al., 1988; Press and Phoenix, 2005; Heide-Jørgenson, 2008). However, parasites vary in their host specificity (Norton and Carpenter, 1998), and even generalists show high levels of host preference. For example, dodder *Cuscuta costaricensis* (Convolvulaceae), is considered to be a generalist with a wide host range, but this species does not use all host plants equally (Kelly et al., 1988), and may disproportionally extract nutrients from different hosts. The host range of most parasitic plants is poorly known and often based on anecdotal sources (Garcia-Franco and Rico-Gray, 1996; Norton and De Lange, 1999; Heide-Jørgenson, 2008), and quantifying host specificity is complicated by the fact that host species may seem to be 'preferred' as an artefact of their abundance, where some hosts are more frequently encountered by the parasite than others (Press and Phoenix, 2005). Host range in holoparasites such as the broomrapes *Orobanche* may have evolved in association with the host life history of its hosts, since host-specialisation in this genus is associated with predictable resources (perennial hosts) and host-generalism with unpredictable resources (annual hosts) (Schneeweiss, 2007). Obligate holoparasites generally show more specific host requirements than facultative hemiparasites (Estabrook and Yoder, 1998), though even the apparently broad host range observed in many hemiparasitic species may in fact be the result of the occurrence of multiple host-specific races (Yoder, 1997).

For many parasitic plants, the perception of host-derived molecules is species-specific, and after seed germination, this recognition process may occur at several levels of haustorial development including initiation, attachment or host penetration (Riopel and Musselman,

1979). All parasitic plants, whether hemiparasitic or holoparasitic, have the capacity to perceive exogenous host-derived signals that control their development (Riopel and Timko, 1995), and it is the variation in these host-derived molecules, along with parasite perception mechanisms, that appear to form the basis of host specificity. Most parasitic plants produce exceptionally minute seeds with small seed reserves, and must attach to a suitable host soon after germination to ensure survival (Shen et al., 2006). Germination of parasitic plant seeds therefore requires specific chemical stimulants called xenognosins produced by host roots (Press et al., 1990; Hauck et al., 1992; Pérez-de-Luque *et al.*, 2000; Goldwasser and Yoder, 2001; Matusova et al., 2005, Awad et al., 2006). Germination stimulants are important determinants of host specificity in some parasitic plants (Shen et al., 2006). In some interactions for example, host specificity is due to the production of different stimulants by host plants (Press et al., 1990), which determines which potential hosts seeds will germinate on.

Following germination, parasitic plant seedlings attach to, and penetrate the epidermis of the host root or stem, and connect with the host vascular system via an intrusive, multicellular haustorium (Press et al., 1991; Riopel and Timko, 1995; Estabrook and Yoder, 1998; Zehhar et al., 2003). The haustorium is a defining phenotypic feature of all parasitic angiosperms (Estabrook and Yoder, 1998; Hibberd and Jeschke, 2001), and importantly provides a vascular conduit between host and parasite, representing a physiological bridge between the two plants (Kuijt, 1969; Riopel and Timko, 1995), through which hormonal interactions are facilitated (Press and Graves, 1995), and viruses, proteins and mRNA transcripts may be transported (David-Schwartz et al., 2008) (Figure 5). The chemical signals involved in initiating haustorial development are distinct from the signals which induce germination (Riopel and Timko, 1995), and are also important determinants of host specificity (Shen et al., 2006). The unique developmental process of haustorium initiation in parasitic angiosperms relies on a suite of specific exogenous molecules in the rhizosphere, called haustoria-inducing factors (HIFs) (Riopel and Timko, 1995). The development of haustoria in parasitic plants can be triggered by multiple host-derived molecules, therefore specific host-parasite interactions at the level of haustorial development adds a further dimension to host specificity.

Even after the successful establishment of host-parasite vascular connectivity, host-resistance responses can abort the development of the parasite. An array of different mechanisms of host resistance to the invasion of the haustorium exist, and can be elicited at different stages in the infection process, resulting in the arrest of parasite development (Boone et al., 1995; Yoder, 1997; Fernández-Aparicio et al., 2009a). Thus, host recognition by parasitic plants follows a series of developmental checkpoints (Yoder, 1997). At the cellular level, variation in response to germination stimulants, HIFs and uncharacterised signals initiating the differentiation of vascular tissue, all appear to contribute to the early stages of host specificity. Parasite development may then elicit host resistance responses, which are quantitative, multigenic characters (Kim et al., 1998) that are the result of several mechanisms acting at different stages of infection by the parasite (Katzir et al., 1996; Pérez-de-Luque et al., 2005).

In summary, host specificity is the consequence of an evolutionary arms race between host and parasite; parasitic plants reduce the fitness of their host associates, therefore selection will favour the most resistant hosts. Conversely attached parasites may be aborted by a multitude of host resistance responses, and selection will favour the most virulent strains that can overcome this resistance. Investigations have not yet explored this important co-evolutionary process in parasitic plants at the combined molecular, physiological and population level, which would clearly be of value from both ecological and agricultural perspectives.

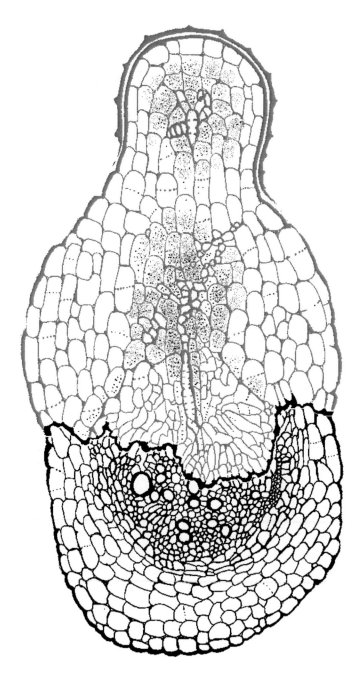

Figure 5. The haustorium of a parasitic plant which provides a vascular conduit and physiological bridge between host and parasite, through which hormonal interactions are facilitated and viruses, proteins and mRNA transcripts may be transported.

HOST SPECIFICITY AS A PROMOTER OF SPECIATION

Host specificity is established to be an important template for speciation in phytophagus insects (McCoy et al., 2001), in which populations of insects become isolated and genetically divergent on host plants with differing ecologies (Funk et al., 1995; Funk et al., 2002). Host-driven speciation is often a consequence of host shifting or "switching", which occurs when a population establishes on a novel host to which it is "preadapted", and then genetically diverges from its precursor population (Futuyma et al., 1994; Norton and De Lange 1999; Drès and Mallet 2002; Funk et al., 2002). Host switching may occur following a change in the abundance of the predominantly infected host species, or if a parasite expands its range and encounters new host species (Norton and Carpenter, 1998). Such host-switching is believed to have been a route to speciation in insects, e.g. leafminers (*Phytomyza* spp.) (Scheffer and Wiegmann, 2000) and walking-sticks (*Timena* spp.) (Crespi and Sandoval 2000). Furthermore, host specificity has the potential to drive the synchronous speciation of parasites with their host associates, producing congruent phylogenies, a relationship referred to as Fahrenholz's rule (Fahrenholz, 1913; Hafner and Nadler 1988; Hafner and Page 1995), for example leaf beetles (*Ophraella* spp.) which have co-speciated with their hosts in the Asteraceae (Funk et al., 1995).

The extent to which host shifts followed by ecological divergence or host-parasite co-evolution have facilitated speciation in parasitic plants is largely unknown. The distribution of parasitic plants is tightly correlated with their host specificities (Heide-Jørgenson, 2008). Many parasites described as host-generalists have, on closer inspection, been shown to be specialists at a local level (Norton and Carpenter, 1998; Thorogood and Hiscock, 2007), suggesting the degree of host specificity in parasites is probably underestimated (Thorogood, 2008). Host specificity may be a precursor to race formation in parasitic plants where gene flow between populations is restricted over time (Norton and Carpenter, 1998), for example if parasite populations are also inbreeding. Given the distinct patterns of host specificity observed in most obligate holoparasitic plants (Estabrook and Yoder, 1998), host-associated divergence is likely to have been an important evolutionary process in these angiosperms. Several studies indicate that host-driven divergence may indeed have been an underestimated driver of speciation in both hemiparasites (Nickrent and Stell 1990; Zuber and Widmer 2000; Jerome and Ford 2002a; Jerome and Ford 2002b) and holoparasites (Thorogood and Hiscock 2007; de Vega et al., 2008; Thorogood et al., 2008, 2009b), and may therefore be a taxonomically widespread phenomenon.

HOST-DRIVEN SPECIATION IN HEMIPARASITIC PLANTS

Most studies on host-driven divergence have been carried out using hemiparasitic mistletoes, a diverse group of stem-parasites in the order Santalales. For example, reciprocal transplant experiments have demonstrated that races of Mistletoe (*Phoradendron tomentosum* [Santalaceae]) are physiologically adapted to particular host trees. Mistletoes that were collected from three different host trees and planted reciprocally onto the branches of these hosts in a natural plant community showed significantly greater haustorial disk development on the natural hosts than on the experimental hosts (Clay et al., 1985). This physiological adaptation to local hosts may have preceded genetic divergence among host-specific races of *Phoradendron*. Nickrent and Stell (1990) first provided evidence for genetic differentiation in two host-races of the hemiparasitic hemlock dwarf mistletoe (*Aeceuthobium tsugense* [Viscaceae]) using electrophoretic isozyme loci. Races were defined by both geographic location and host range, yet they were morphologically indistinguishable. Host range is believed to have played a major role in providing potential niches for parasite colonisation in the *Aeceuthobium* genus, in which rapid adaptive radiations onto numerous host tree species may have obscured more profound levels of population differentiation at the molecular level (Nickrent and Butler, 1991; Nickrent, 2002). Similarly, Jerome and Ford (2002a, 2002b) identified genetic races of the dwarf mistletoe *A. americanum* in a molecular analysis using amplified fragment length polymorphism (AFLP) loci in North America and Canada. As previously identified in *A. tsugense* (Nickrent and Stell 1990), genetic differentiation in *A. americanum* was associated with geographic isolation as well as host range. Therefore host identity, isolation-by-distance, and environmental parameters collectively appear to have contributed to the evolution of genetic races in the mistletoe genus *Aeceuthobium*.

Host specificity has been the basis for the taxonomic classification of *Viscum album* (Viscaceae) in Northern Europe, in which four morphologically indistinguishable subspecies are apparently physiologically adapted to different species of host. The commonest subspecies *V. album* spp. *album* has been recorded to infect more than 230 species of tree from over 100 genera (Heide-Jørgenson, 2008) and can clearly be considered a host generalist. However *V. album* spp. *abietis* is specific to the coniferous genus *Abies*, *V. album* spp. *astriacum* is restricted to *Pinus* spp. and *Larix* spp., and *V. album* spp. *cruciatum* (also recognized at the specific rank), grows preferentially on *Olea europaea* (Ball, 1993). Evidence from chloroplast DNA (cpDNA) and nuclear DNA internal transcribed spacer (nDNA ITS) sequence data support the separation of these taxa into distinct genetic races (Zuber and Widmer 2000), despite their cryptic morphology. Host specificity is also a feature of mistletoes in the Loranthaceae (Norton and deLange, 1999), and may therefore be a widespread precursor to speciation among host-races in mistletoes generally (Norton and Carpenter, 1998).

Few studies have investigated host-driven population differentiation in hemiparasites besides mistletoes, however this pattern has been reported for populations of the hemiparasitic weedy species *Striga gesnerioides* (Orobanchaceae), parasitising host species *Indigofera hirsuta* and *Vigna ungiculata* in Central Florida and West Africa, using AFLP marker data (Botanga and Timko, 2005).

HOST-DRIVEN SPECIATION IN HOLOPARASITIC PLANTS

Little work has focused on speciation in holoparasites, but given that obligate holoparasites often show greater host specificity than facultative hemiparasites (Estabrook and Yoder, 1998), they might be expected to be strongly predisposed to host-driven speciation. *Cytinus* spp. (Cytinaceae, ex-Rafflesiaceae) are endophytic holoparasites that occur in the Mediterranean Basin and South Africa and have recently been classified as sister to Muntingiaceae (Nickrent, 2007), an American family of woody shrubs. These holoparasites are morphologically cryptic, and show host specificity at both a local and regional scale

(Thorogood and Hiscock, 2007; deVega et al., 2008). For example, *Cytinus hypocistis* has been found to be locally host-specific in the Algarve region of Portugal where only two hosts in the Cistaceae were consistently infected: *Halimium halimifolium* and *Cistus monspeliensis*. *Cytinus hypocistis* did not infect hosts in proportion to their abundance; at three sites, 100% of parasites occurred on *H. halimifolium* which represented just 42.4%, 3% and 19.7% of potential hosts available, and at the remaining site in the absence of *H. halimifolium,* 100% of parasites occurred on *C. monspeliensis*. Other species of potential host were consistently uninfected irrespective of their abundance (Thorogood and Hiscock, 2007). Such patterns of host specificity at a local level may contribute to the partitioning of genetic diversity on a regional scale. For example a recent molecular marker-based investigation identified five genetic races of *Cytinus sensu lato* in the Mediterranean Basin, which were associated with infrageneric sections of host species in the Cistaceae (deVega et al., 2008). This AFLP-based study identified genetic races of *Cytinus* that preferentially infect, respectively, species of *Cistus* sect. *Ladanium*, *Cistus* sect. *Ledonia*, *Cistus* sect. *Cistus*, and *Halimium* sect. *Chrysorhodion*. Such a pattern of host-driven genetic divergence with restricted gene flow between cryptic races had not previously been reported for parasitic angiosperms. Differentiation of genera in the Cistaceae occurred during the Oligocene to Miocene, which suggests that the *Cytinus*–Cistaceae association has undergone a long period of evolutionary divergence, reinforcing adaptation of *Cytinus* to different host species. This study investigated the genetic variability of *Cytinus* in SW Spain and Morocco, however given this species *sensu lato* is a circum-Mediterranean complex, to resolve taxonomic relationships in relation to host specificity, a regional-scale study must be carried out.

Host-associated radiations may also have occurred in the genus *Orobanche* (Orobanchaceae). The genus *Orobanche* comprises over 150 described species of root holoparasite, the majority of which occur in the Mediterranean region of Europe, Asia Minor and North Africa. Holoparasitism has led to reductions in gross morphological features in *Orobanche* traditionally used in plant classification, for example the loss of lack true leaves and roots (Román *et al.,* 2007) and they comprise a taxonomically challenging genus (Rumsey and Jury 1991; Plaza et al., 2004). Recent attempts to analyse the phylogenetic relationships in the genus *Orobanche* have used conventional markers such as nuclear internal transcribed spacer (ITS), plastid *rbcL,* and *rps2* gene sequences (Manen et al., 2004; Schneeweiss et al., 2004; Park et al., 2008). However, these investigations failed to resolve the relationships among the more closely related species of *Orobanche*, especially those within the taxonomically difficult *Minores* complex. Species in this species complex are host-specific but morphologically similar, suggesting that cryptic host-specific taxa may be genetically isolated by the distinct ecologies of their different host species. Such patterns of ecological isolation may, ultimately, provide a template for speciation. Most *Orobanche* species have a very narrow host range (Schneeweiss, 2007), however some taxa are more-or-less restricted to a single host species for example: *O. serbica* on *Artemisia alba; O. lucorum* on *Berberis vulgaris;* and *O. laserpitii-sileris* on *Laserpitium siler* (Thorogood, 2008). On the other hand, a few species have evolved a very broad host range, for example *O. minor,* which parasitizes a diverse range of angiosperms from at least 16 orders in both the monocots and eudicots (CJ Thorogood unpublished data). Specialization to particular hosts among host-generalist species may have contributed to the taxonomic complexity of this systematically challenging genus.

Host race differentiation has been identified in populations of the weedy species *O. foetida* growing on either chickpea and faba bean, which is speculated to be a result of strong selection following adaptation to these commercial host species (Román *et al.*, 2007). Given that host-races of *O. foetida* respond differently to germination stimulants produced by chickpea and faba bean respectively, specificity may be selected for at the stage of germination in this species. Evidence suggests that natural *O. foetida* also show genotypic differentiation among natural host-specific populations (Vaz Patto et al., 2007). Studying host specificity in natural populations of weedy species may be an important approach to understanding the process of host-shifting from natural species to commercial crops in parasitic plants such as *Orobanche*.

Molecular markers have also identified host-associated genetic divergence between natural populations of intraspecific taxa *O. minor* var. *minor* and *O. minor* ssp. *maritima* associated with either Red Clover (*Trifolium pratense*) or Sea Carrot (*Daucus carota* ssp. *gummifer*) respectively, in Northern Europe (Thorogood et al., 2008). *Orobanche minor* ssp. *maritima* (previously ranked at the varietal level) shows marked host specificity, and grows preferentially on *Daucus carota* ssp. *gummifer* (Apiaceae), and more rarely on *Plantago coronopus* (Plantaginaceae) (Rumsey, 1994). The distribution of *O. minor* ssp. *maritima* is correlated with its host range and it favours steep, calcareous grassland on south-facing sea cliffs. *Orobanche minor* var. *minor* however, has been introduced in seed mixes throughout much of its British range (Rumsey, 2007) and occurs on a wide range of host species from taxonomically disparate families, often on disturbed or cultivated sites (Rumsey and Jury 1991). Inter-simple sequence repeat markers (ISSRs) provided evidence of host-driven divergence between populations, which was supported by phylogenetic analyses based on sequence-characterised amplified region (SCAR)-based sequence data. While molecular data indicated genetic differentiation, populations appeared to be poorly differentiated morphologically, suggesting cryptic genetic races may be adapted to local hosts. *Orobanche minor* var. *minor* has a wide host range, and is a pest in some areas, for example on clover crops in the Pacific Northwest of the United States (Eizenberg et al., 2003; Ross et al., 2004). *Orobanche minor* subsp. *maritima* however is nationally scarce in the UK, and highly host-specific (Rumsey, 2007). The difference in host specificity of these weedy and non-weedy infraspecific respectively, supports suggestions that a wide host range in parasitic plants such as *Orobanche* may predispose species or infraspecific races to a weedy life history (Schneeweiss, 2007; Fernández-Aparicio et al., 2009b).

Cross infection studies have confirmed that races of *O. minor* are physiologically adapted to their local hosts (Thorogood et al., 2009). Genetic races of *O. minor* (identified by Thorogood et al., 2008) have been reciprocally cultivated with their natural host species in Petri dish bioassays to quantify the early stages of the infection and establishment processes. In this study, parasite fitness was determined in terms of biomass, and the anatomy of the host-parasite interface investigated using histochemical techniques, to compare the infection process on different hosts. The genetic races showed distinct patterns of host specificity, and yielded a higher fitness on their natural hosts, indicating adaptation to local hosts. In addition, histological evidence suggested that clover and carrot roots vary in their responses to infection, therefore root anatomy and responses to infection may underpin a physiological basis for host specificity in *Orobanche*. Such cross-infection experiments are often time-consuming and difficult to perform (Rumsey and Jury 1991; Zuber and Widmer 2000), however they are useful for demonstrating host specificity (Clay et al., 1985). Many holoparasitic angiosperms are experimentally intractable, owing to their extremely specialized life histories, and specific host ranges. However the rapid life cycle of, for example, *O. minor* (approximately 16 weeks), and its broad host range make this species an ideal model with which to study host-parasite interactions using an experimentally tractable holoparasite. Future studies will investigate host specificity using a combined approach, in which host-parasite interactions are characterised histologically at the cellular level, in conjunction with molecular markers to identify genetic divergence at the population level. This combined approach shows promise as a powerful tool for understanding the mechanisms that underpin host-associated patterns of speciation in parasitic plants.

CONCLUSION

Parasitic plants include some of the great enigmas of the plant world, and yet surprisingly little is known about their evolutionary biology. In natural ecosystems, parasitic plants act as keystone species because they drive shifts in the competitive balance between host and non-host species, thereby altering plant community structure (Press and Phoenix, 2005). Some species of parasitic plant also pose severe problems for agriculture where species have shifted from their natural hosts to commercial crops (Parker and Riches, 1993). Thus parasitic flowering plants are important from evolutionary, ecological and economic perspectives.

Recent advances in molecular phylogenetic techniques, coupled with improved sampling, are now providing the first clear insights into the phylogenetic relationships among holoparasites and their photosynthetic ancestors. However progress in understanding the evolution of speciation in parasitic plants remains comparatively elusive. Speciation in parasitic plants has, until recently, remained a relatively unexplored topic in evolutionary biology, and the understanding of host specificity as a potential catalyst for speciation in these plants has lagged behind that of other organisms such as plant pathogens and phytophagus insects. Nevertheless, recent research into a handful of hemiparasites and holoparasites has provided strong preliminary evidence for host-driven speciation in both hemiparasitic and holoparasitic plants.

These plants show promise as models for studying host-associated speciation processes. Parasitism in these plants ranges from facultative hemiparasitism to obligate holoparasitism, and host specificity ranges from the infection of single host associates to hundreds of species from taxonomically diverse families. Investigations that adopt an integrated approach from the cellular to the ecosystem level in experimentally tractable parasitic plants will offer important insights into the evolution of this economically and ecologically important group of angiosperms.

REFERENCES

APG, 2003. An update of the angiosperm phylogeny group classification for the orders and families of flowering plants: APG II. *Botanical Journal of the Linnaean Society.* 141: 399-436.

Awad AA, Sato D, Kusumoto D, Kamioka H, Takeuchi Y, Yoneyama K. 2006. Characterization of strigolactones, germination stimulants for the root parasitic plants *Striga* and *Orobanche,* produced by maize, millet and sorghum. *Plant Growth Regulation,* 48: 221-227.

Ball PW, 1993. *Viscum* L. In: Flora Europaea, 1: 86 Tutin TG, Burges NA, Chater AO, Edmondson JR, Heywood VH, Moore DM, Valentine DH Walters, SM Webb DA. eds. Flora Europaea, 1: 86, *Cambridge University Press*, Cambridge.

Barkman TJ, Lim S-H, Mat Selleh K, Nais, J, 2004. Mitochondrial DNA sequences reveal the photosynthetic relatives of *Rafflesia*, the world's largest flower. *Proceedings of the National Academy of Sciences USA.* 101: 787-792.

Barkman TJ, McNeal JR, Lim S-H, Coat G, Croom HB, Young ND, dePamphilis CW, 2007. Mitochondrial DNA suggests at least 11 origins of parasitism in angiosperms and reveals genomic chimerism in parasitic plants. *BMC Evolutionary Biology*, 7:248.

Boone LS, Fate G, Chang, M, Lynn DG, 1995. *In* Parasitic plants, Press MC, Graves JD, Eds. Chapman and Hall, London, pp. 14-38.

Botanga CJ, Timko MP, 2005. Genetic structure and analysis of host and nonhost interactions of *Striga gesnerioides* (witchweed) from Central Florida. *Phytopathology*, 95: 1166–1173.

Bungard RA, 2004. Photosynthetic evolution in parasitic plants: insight from the chloroplast genome. *BioEssays*, 26: 235-247.

Callaway RM, Pennings SC, 1998. Impact of a parasitic plant on the zonation of two salt marsh perennials. *Oecologia*, 114:100-105.

Cameron DD, Hwangbo J-K, Keith AM, Geniez J-M, Kraushaar D, Rowntree J, Seel WE, 2005. Interactions between the hemiparasitic angiosperm *Rhinanthus minor* and its hosts: from the cell to the ecosystem. *Folia geobotanica*, 40: 217-229.

Cameron DD, Coats AM, Seel WE, 2006. Differential resistance among host and non-host species underlies the variable success of the hemi-parasitic plant *Rhinanthus minor. Annals of Botany,* 98: 1289-1299.

Cameron DD, Geniez J-M, Seel WE, Irving LJ, 2008. Suppression of host photosynthesis by the parasitic plant *Rhinanthus minor. Annals of Botany*, 101: 573 - 578.

Clay K, Dement D, Rejmanek M, 1985. Experimental evidence for host races in mistletoe (*Phoradendron tormentosum*). *American Journal of Botany*, 72: 1225–1231.

Crespi BJ, Sandoval CP, 2000. Phylogenetic evidence for the evolution of ecological specialization in *Timena* walking-sticks. *Journal of Evolutionary Biology,* 13: 249-262.

Cronquist A, 1988. The evolution and classification of flowering plants. *The New York Botanical Garden,* New York, USA.

David-Schwartz R, Runo S, Townsley B, Machuka J, Sinha N, 2008. Long-distance transport of mRNA via parenchyma cells and phloem across the host–parasite junction in *Cuscuta*. New Phytologist, 179: 1133–1141.

Davies DM, Graves, JD, Elias CO, Williams PJ, 1997. The impact of *Rhinanthus* spp. on sward productivity and composition: implications for the restoration of species-rich *grasslands. Biological Conservation,* 82: 87-93.

Davis CC, Latvis M, Nickrent DL, Wurdack KJ, Baum DA, 2007. Floral gigantism in Rafflesiaceae. *Science*, 315: 1812.

Davis CC, Wurdack KJ, 2004. Host-to-parasite gene transfer in flowering plants: phylogenetic evidence from Malpighiales. *Science*, 303: 676-678.

Davis CC, 2008. Floral evolution: dramatic size change was recent and rapid in the world's largest flowers. *Current Biology*, 18: 1102-1104.

dePamphilis CW, Palmer JD, 1990. Loss of photosynthetic and chlororespiratory genes from the plastid genome of a parasitic flowering plant. *Nature*, 348: 337-339.

dePamphilis CW, 1995. In Press MC, Graves JD, Eds. Parasitic plants. *Chapman and Hall*, London, pp. 177-205.

dePamphilis CW, Young ND, Wolfe AD, 1997. Evolution of plastid gene *rps2* in a lineage of hemiparasitic and holoparasitic plants: many losses of photosynthesis and complex patterns of rate variation. *Proceedings of the National Academy of Sciences*, 94: 7367-7372.

deVega C, Berjano R, Arista M, Ortiz PL, Talavera S, Stuessy TF, 2008. Genetic races associated with the genera and sections of host species in the holoparasitic plant *Cytinus* (Cytinaceae) in the Western Mediterranean basin. *New Phytologist*, 178: 875–887.

Drès M, Mallet J, 2002. Host races in plant-feeding insects and their importance in sympatric speciation. *Philosophical Transactions of the Royal Society of London Series B*, 357: 471–492.

Eizenberg H, Colquhoun JB, Mallory-Smith CA, 2003. Variation in clover response to small broomrape (*Orobanche minor*). *Weed Science*, 51: 759-763.

Estabrook EM, Yoder JI, 1998. Plant-plant communications: rhizosphere signaling between parasitic angiosperms and their hosts. *Plant Physiology*, 116: 1-7.

Fahrenholz H, 1913. Ectoparasiten und abstammungslehre. *Zoologischer Anzeiger*, 41: 371–374.

Fernández-Aparicio M, Sillero JC, Rubiales D, 2009a. Resistance to broomrape species (*Orobanche* spp.) in common vetch (*Vicia sativa* L.). *Crop Protection*, 28: 7-12.

Fernández-Aparicio M, Flores F, Rubiales D, 2009b. Recognition of root exudates by seeds of broomrape (*Orobanche* and *Phelipanche*) species. *Annals of Botany*, 103: 423 - 431.

Funk DJ, Futuyma DJ, Ortí G, Meyer A, 1995. A history of host associations and evolutionary diversification for *Ophraella* (Coleoptera: Chrysomelidae): new evidence from mitochondrial DNA. *Evolution*, 49: 1008–1017.

Funk DJ, Filchak KE, Feder JL, 2002. Herbivorous insects: model systems for the comparative study of speciation ecology. *Genetica*, 116: 251–267.

Futuyma DJ, Walsh JS, Morton T, Funk DJ, Keese MC, 1994. Genetic variation in a phylogenetic context: responses of two specialized leaf beetles (Coleoptera: Chrysomelidae) to host plants of their congeners. *Journal of Evolutionary Biology*,: 7: 127-146.

Garcia-Franco JG, Rico-Gray V, 1996. Distribution and host specificity in the holoparasite *Bdallophyton bambusarum* (Rafflesiaceae) in a tropical deciduous forest in Veracruz, Mexico. *Biotropica*, 28: 759-762.

Gibson CC, Watkinson AR, 1989. The host range and selectivity of a parasitic plant – *Rhinanthus minor* L. *Oecologia*, 78: 401-406.

Goldwasser Y, Yoder JI. 2001. Differential induction of *Orobanche* seed germination by *Arabidopsis thaliana*. *Plant Science* 160: 951-959.

Hafner MS, Nadler SA, 1988. Phylogenetic trees support the coevolution of parasites and their hosts. *Nature*, 332: 258– 259.

Hafner MS, Page RDM, 1995. Molecular phylogenies and host-parasite cospeciation: gophers and lice as a model system. *Philosophical Transactions of the Royal Society B*, 349: 77–83.

Hauck C, Muller S, Schildknecht H, 1992. A germination stimulant for the parasitic flowering plants from *Sorghum bicolour,* a genuine host plant. *Journal of Plant Physiology,* 139: 474-478.

Heide-Jørgenson HS, 2008. Parasitic flowering plants. *Brill,* Boston.

Hibberd JM, Quick, WP, Press MC, Scholes JD, Jeschke WD, 1999. Solute fluxes from tobacco to the parasitic angiosperm *Orobanche cernua* and the influence of infection on host carbon and nitrogen relations. *Plant, Cell and Environment,* 22: 937–947.

Hibberd JM, Jeschke WD, 2001. Solute flux into parasitic plants. *Journal of Experimental Botany,* 52: 2043-2049.

Jerome CA, Ford BA, 2002a. The discovery of three genetic races of the dwarf mistletoe *Arceuthobium americanum* (Viscaceae) provides insight into the evolution of parasitic angiosperms. *Molecular Ecology* 11: 387-405.

Jerome CA, Ford BA, 2002b. Comparative population structure and genetic diversity of *Arceuthobium americanum* (Viscaceae) and its *Pinus* host species: insight into host-parasite evolution in parasitic angiosperms. *Molecular Ecology,* 11: 407-420.

Jones CG, Lawton JH, Shachak M, 1994. Organisms as ecosystem engineers. *Oikos,* 69: 373-386.

Katzir N, Portnoy V, Tzuri G, Castejon-Munoz M, Joel DM. 1996. Use of amplified polymorphic DNA (RAPD) markers in the study of the parasitic weed *Orobanche. Theoretical and applied genetics* 93: 367-372.

Kelly CK, Venable DL, Zimmerer K. 1988. Host specialization in *Cuscuta costaricensis*: an assessment of host use relative to host availability. *Oikos,* 53: 315-320.

Kim D, Kocz R, Boone L, Keyes WJ and Lynn DG. 1998. On becoming a parasite: evaluating the role of wall oxidases in parasitic plant development. *Chemistry and Biology,* 5: 103-117.

Kuijt J, 1969. The biology of parasitic flowering plants. *University of California Press,* Berkeley.

Manen JF, Habashi C, Jeanmonod D, Park JM, Schneeweiss GM, 2004. Phylogeny and intraspecific variability of holoparasitic *Orobanche* (Orobanchaceae) inferred from plastid *rbcL* sequences. *Molecular Phylogenetics and Evolution,* 33: 482–500.

Marvier MA, 1998. Parasite impacts on host communities: plant parasitism in a California coastal prairie. *Ecology,* 79: 2616–2623.

Matusova R, Rani K, Verstappen FWA, Franssen MCR, Beale MH, Bouwmeester HJ, 2005. The strigolactone germination stimulants of the plant-parasitic *Striga* and *Orobanche* ssp. are derived from the carotenoid pathway. *Plant Physiology,* 139: 920-934.

McCoy KD, Boulinier T, Tirard C, Michalakis Y, 2001. Host specificity of a generalist parasite: genetic evidence of sympatric host races in the seabird tick *Ixodes uriae. Journal of Evolutionary Biology,* 14: 395-405.

Molau, U 1995. In Press MC, Graves JD, Eds. Parasitic plants. *Chapman and Hall,* London, pp. 141-176.

Musselman LJ and Press MC, 1995. In Press MC, Graves JD, Eds. Parasitic plants. *Chapman and Hall,* London, pp. 141-176.

Nais J, 2001. *Rafflesia* of the world. Sabah Parks, Kota Kinabalu.

Nickrent DL Stell AL, 1990. Biochemical systematics of the *Arceuthobium campylopodum* complex (dwarf mistletoes, Viscaceae). II. Electrophoretic evidence for genetic differentiation in two host races of hemlock dwarf mistletoe (*A. tsugense*). *Biochemical Systematics and Ecology,* 18: 267-280.

Nickrent DL, Butler TL, 1991. Genetic Relationships in *Arceuthobium monticola* and *A. siskiyouense* (Viscaceae): New Dwarf Mistletoe Species from California and Oregon. *Biochemical Systematics and Ecology*, 19: 305-313.

Nickrent DL, Blarer A, Qiu Y-L, Soltis DE, Soltis PS, Zanis M, 2002. Molecular data place Hydnoraceae with Aristolochiaceae. *American Journal of Botany*, 89: 1809-1817.

Nickrent DL, Blarer A, Qiu Y-L, Vidal-Russell R, Anderson FE, 2004. Phylogenetic inference in Rafflesiales: the influence of rate heterogeneity and horizontal gene transfer. *BMC Evolutionary Biology*, 4: 40.

Nickrent DL, Der JP, Anderson FE, 2005. Discovery of the photosynthetic relatives of the "Maltese mushroom" *Cynomorium. BMC Evolutionary Biology*, 5:38.

Nickrent DL, 2007. Cytinaceae are sister to Muntingiaceae (Malvales). *Taxon*, 56: 1129–1135.

Norton DA, Carpenter MA. 1998. Mistletoes as parasites: host specificity and speciation. *Trends in Ecology and Evolution*, 13: 101-105.

Norton DA, De Lange PJ. 1999. Host specificity in parasitic mistletoes (Loranthaceae) in New Zealand. *Functional Ecology* 13: 552-559.

Park J-M Manen J-F Colwell AE Schneeweiss GM, 2008. A plastid gene phylogeny of the non-photosynthetic parasitic *Orobanche* (Orobanchaceae) and related genera. Journal of Plant Research 121: 365–376.

Parker C, Riches CR. 1993. Parasitic weeds of the world – biology and control. Wallingford, *CABI publishing*, Oxford.

Pate JS, 1995. In Parasitic plants. Press MC, Graves JD, Eds. *Chapman and Hall*, London, pp. 80-102.

Pérez-de-Luque A, Galindo JCG, Macias FA, Jorrin J. 2000. Sunflower sesquiterpene lactone models induce *Orobanche cumana* seed germination. *Phytochemistry* 53: 45-50.

Pérez-de-Luque A, Rubiales D, Cubero JI, Press MC, Scholes J, Yoneyama K, Takeuchi Y, Plakhine D and Joel DM, 2005. Interaction between *Orobanche crenata* and its host legumes: unsuccessful haustorial penetration and necrosis of the developing parasite. *Annals of Botany*, 95: 935-942.

Phoenix GK, Press MC, 2005. Linking physiological traits to impacts on community structure and function: the role of root hemiparasitic Orobanchaceae (ex-Scrophulariaceae). *Journal of Ecology*, 93: 67-78.

Plaza L, Fernández I, Juan R, Pastor J, Pujadas A, 2004. Micromorphological studies on seeds of *Orobanche* species from the Iberian peninsula and the Balearic Islands, and their systematic significance. *Annals of Botany,* 94: 167-178.

Press MC, Graves JD, and Stewart GR, 1990. Physiology of the interaction of angiosperm parasites and their higher plant hosts. *Plant, Cell and Environment,* 13: 91-104.

Press MC, Smith S, and Stewart GR, 1991. Carbon acquisition and assimilation in parasitic plants. *Functional Ecology* 5: 278-283.

Press MC, Graves JD. 1995. Parasitic plants. *Chapman and Hall,* London.

Press MC, 1998. Dracula or Robin Hood? A functional role for root hemiparasites in nutrient poor ecosystems. *Oikos*, 82: 609-611.

Press MC, Phoenix GK, 2005. Impacts of parasitic plants on natural communities. *New Phytologist* 166: 737-751.

Quested HM, Press MC, Callaghan TV, Cornelissen JHC, 2001. The hemiparasitic angiosperm *Bartsia alpina* has the potential to accelerate decomposition in sub-arctic communities. *Oecologia*, 130: 88–95.

Quested HM, 2008. Parasitic plants-impacts on nutrient cycling. *Plant and Soil*, 311: 269-272.

Randle CP, Wolfe AD. 2005. The evolution and expression of *RBCL* in holoparasitic sister-genera *Harveya* and *Hyobanche* (Orobanchaceae). *American Journal of Botany*, 92: 1575-1585.

Riopel JL, Musselman LJ, 1979. Experimental Initiation of Haustoria in *Agalinis purpurea* (Scrophulariaceae). *American Journal of Botany*, 66: 570-575.

Riopel JL, Timko MP, 1995. In Parasitic plants. Press MC, Graves JD, Eds. *Chapman and Hall*, London, pp. 39-79.

Román B, Satovic Z, Alfaro C, Moreno MT, Kharrat M, Pérez-de-Luque A, Rubiales D, 2007. Host differentiation in *Orobanche foetida* Poir. *Flora*, 202: 201–208.

Ross KC, Colquhoun JB, Mallory-Smith CA, 2004. Small broomrape (*Orobanche minor*) germination and early development in response to plant species. *Weed Science*, 52: 260-266.

Rumsey FJ, 1994. *Orobanche minor* var. *maritima* In Stewart A, Pearman DA, Preston CD, Eds. Scarce plants in Britain. *J. N. C. C.* Peterborough.

Rumsey FJ, 2007. A reconsideration of *Orobanche maritima* Pugsley (Orobanchaceae) and related taxa in southern England and the Channel Islands. *Watsonia*, 26: 473-476.

Rumsey FJ, Jury SL, 1991. An account of *Orobanche* L. in Britain and Ireland. *Watsonia*, 18: 257-295.

Scheffer SJ, Wiegmann BM, 2000. Molecular Phylogenetics of the Holly Leafminers (Diptera: Agromyzidae: *Phytomyza*): Species Limits, Speciation, and Dietary Specialization. *Molecular Phylogenetics and Evolution*, 17: 244-255.

Schneeweiss GM, Colwell A, Park J-M, Jang C-G, Stuessy TF, 2004. Phylogeny of holoparasitic *Orobanche* (Orobanchaceae) inferred from nuclear ITS sequences. *Molecular Phylogenetics and Evolution*, 30: 465–478.

Schneeweiss GM, 2007. Correlated evolution of life history and host range in the nonphotosynthetic parasitic flowering plants *Orobanche* and *Phelipanche* (Orobanchaceae). *Journal of Evolutionary Biology*, 20: 471–478.

Searcy DG, 1970. Measurements by DNA hybridisation *in vitro* of the genetic basis of parasite reductions. *Evolution*, 24: 207-219.

Searcy DG, MacInnis AJ, 1970. Measurements by DNA renaturation of the genetic basis of parasite reduction. *Evolution*, 24: 796-806.

Shen H, Ye W, Hong L, Huang H, Wang Z, Deng X, Yang Q,. Xu Z, 2006. Progress in Parasitic Plant Biology: Host Selection and Nutrient Transfer. *Plant Biology*, 8: 175–185.

Takhtajan A, 1997. Diversity and Classification of flowering plants. Columbia University Press, New York ,USA.

Thorogood CJ, Hiscock SJ, 2007. Host Specificity in the Parasitic Plant *Cytinus hypocistis*. *Research Letters in Ecology*: 84234.

Thorogood CJ, 2008. Host specificity and speciation in parasitic plants. *Haustorium*, 54: 1-3.

Thorogood CJ, Rumsey FJ, Harris SA, Hiscock SJ, 2008. Host-driven divergence in the parasitic plant *Orobanche minor* Sm. (Orobanchaceae). *Molecular Ecology*, 17: 4289–4303.

Thorogood CJ, Rumsey FJ, Hiscock SJ, 2009. Host-specific races in the holoparasitic angiosperm *Orobanche minor*: implications for speciation in parasitic plants. *Annals of Botany*, in Press.

Vaz Patto MC, Díaz-Ruiz R, Satovic Z, Román B, Pujadas-Salvà AJ, Rubiales D, 2008. Genetic diversity of Moroccan populations of *Orobanche foetida*: evolving from parasitising wild hosts to crop plants. *Weed Research* 48, 179-186.

Wimpee CF, Wrobel RL, Garvin DK, 1991. A divergent plastid genome in *Conopholis americana*, an achlorophyllous parasitic plant. *Plant Molecular Biology*, 17: 161-166.

Wolfe AD, dePamphilis CW, 1998. The effect of relaxed functional constraints on the photosynthetic gene *rbcL* in photosynthetic and nonphotosynthetic parasitic plants. *Molecular Biology and Evolution*, 15: 1243-1258.

Yoder JI, 1997. A species-specific recognition system directs haustorium development in the parasitic plant *Triphysaria* (Scrophulariaceae). *Planta* 202: 407-413.

Young ND, Steiner KE, dePamphilis CW, 1999. The evolution of parasitism in Scrophulariaceae/Orobanchaceae: plastid gene sequences refute evolutionary transition series. *Annals of the Missouri Botanical Garden,* 86: 876-893.

Zehhar N, Labrousse P, Arnaud M-C, Boulet C, Bouya I, Fer A. 2003. Study of resistance to *Orobanche ramosa* in host (oilseed rape and carrot) and non-host (maize) plants. *European Journal of Plant Pathology*, 109: 75-82.

Zuber D, Widmer A, 2000. Genetic evidence for host specificity in the hemi-parasitic *Viscum album* L. (Viscaceae). *Molecular Ecology*, 9: 1069–1073.

In: Phylogeography
Editor: Damien S. Rutgers

Chapter 4

GENE FLOW, GENETIC DRIFT, AND GEOGRAPHIC VARIATION OF THE AINU: AN ASSESSMENT BASED ON NONMETRIC CRANIAL TRAITS

Tsunehiko Hanihara[*]

Department of Anatomy and Biological Anthropology,
Saga Medical School, Saga, Japan

ABSTRACT

Gene flow and genetic drift are important factors affecting geographic variation of human phenotypic traits. In the present study, the effects of gene flow from an outside source on the pattern of within- and among-group variation of Hokkaido Ainu, one of the most generalized eastern Asian populations, are examined by applying R-matrix method to 24 nonmetric cranial traits. The R-matrix method is developed initially for single-locus traits and modified for use with quantitative (metric) phenotypic data. In this study, tetrachoric correlation coefficients estimated by maximum likelihood method, the threshold value for each trait estimated by univariate probit analysis, and the census population sizes of the regional groups of the recent Ainu were used for applying the R-matrix method to nonmetric morphological data. Within-group variance based on nonmetric data was estimated by bootstrap sampling method. The results obtained suggest the possibility of admixture between the immigrants from Northeast Asia as represented by the Okhotsk culture people and the indigenous inhabitants in Hokkaido during the 5th – 12th centuries A.D., at least in the coastal region along the Sea of Okhotsk. Such gene flow from Northeast Asian continent may have a certain degree of effect on genetic structure of recent Ainu as suggested from morphological and ancient mitochondrial DNA evidence. The present findings suggest, moreover, a possible inter-population relationship between the Ainu and non-Ainu Japanese at recent period of time. The present analyses provide results that can be interpreted in terms of archaeologically and historically suggested pattern of gene flow and isolation.

* Correspondence to: Tsunehiko Hanihara
Department of Anatomy and Biological Anthropology, Saga Medical School,
Nabeshima, Saga 849-8501, Japan
E-mail: hanihara@cc.saga-u.ac.jp

Keywords: Okhotsk culture people, Japanese, Northeast Asia, R-matrix method, population
structure

INTRODUCTION

Recent investigations have shown that geographic distance is one of the significant and
primary determinant factors for genetic as well as phenotypic variation and diversification on
both local and global levels (Relethford; 1996, 2004a, b; 2008; Eller, 1999; Serre and Pääbo,
2004; Manica et al., 2005, 2007; Prugnolle et al., 2005; Ramachandran et al., 2005; Liu et al.,
2006; Hanihara, 2008; Von Cramon-Taubadel and Lycett, 2008; Betti et al., 2009). However,
modern human variation and the processes that gave rise to such variation are linked more or
less with the adaptation to local environment including subsistence pattern, the process of
demographic expansion of populations, migration as well as admixture, isolation, or
combination of these factors (Relethford and Blangero, 1990; Lahr, 1996). Migration can
change patterns of intra- and intergroup variation through the action of gene flow, primarily
by increasing variation within groups and decreasing genetic difference between groups,
except possibly for kin-structured migration (Fix, 1978; Relethford, 1991). Migration is,
therefore, additional research focus in the studies of population history and structure
(Relethford and Harpending, 1994; Relethford, 2004b).

Concerning the population history and structure of the Japanese including Ainu, the "dual
structure model" (Hanihara, 1991) is generally held. According to this model, modern
Japanese have two primary origins: the aboriginal Jomon, Neolithic hunter-gatherers, and
migrants from the eastern Asian continent via the Korean Peninsula to the southwestern part
of Japan, who brought rice agriculture and metalworking technologies. During the period
from the end of the Jomon age to the early historic age, or from 2,300 years B.P. to 1,300
years B.P., admixture between the indigenous Jomon people and the incoming populations
blurred the distinction between the two populations except for geographically isolated
Hokkaido. The impact of the post-Jomon migrants was unexpectedly large, so that the
majority of modern Japanese carry a large amount of eastern Asian characteristics (Hanihara,
1991; Hammer and Horai, 1995; Horai et al., 1996; Omoto, 1995; Omot and Saitou, 1997;
Hanihara et al., 1998, 2008; Hanihara and Ishida, 2009). On the other hand, Ainu retain
several archaic characteristic which can be traced back to those of the Neolithic Jomon
population. The Ainu, the indigenous inhabitants of Hokkaido, are an ethnic group with a
distinct Ainu culture appeared at early 14th century A.D.

During the period of 1,500 – 800 years B.P., the Okhotsk culture reached from the
northernmost part of Hokkaido through the coastal region of the Sea of Okhotsk to eastern
Hokkaido (Ishida, 1994, 1995; 1996; Hanihara et al., 2008). The people of the Okhotsk
culture shared physical and cultural characteristics with the populations in the lower basin of
the Amur River such as Nivkhi, Orochs, Ulchs, Nanaians, Negidals, etc. (Ishida1996;
Hudson, 2004; Tajima et al., 2004; Sato et al., 2007, 2009; Komesu et al., 2008). The recent
studies suggest that gene flow from Northeast Asia has certain degree of effect on the genetic
structure of the recent Ainu in Hokkaido (Kondo, 2004; Shigematsu et al., 2004; Hanihara et
al., 2008; Sato et al., 2009). Nevertheless, phenotypic features of recent Ainu are more or less
different from those of the neighboring populations such as continental East/Northeast Asians

and non-Ainu Japanese (Yamaguchi, 1982, 1992; Turner, 1987, 1990; Brace and Hunt, 1990; Dodo and Ishida, 1990). Although many studies of biological variation across the Japanese archipelago have provided several lines of evidence that are related to population history of Japanese (reviewed by Hanihara, 1991), the relationship between Ainu and the neighboring populations as viewed from population structure are still controversial and focus of debate.

Standard multivariate approaches so far been performed in morphological analyses, such as Mahalanobis' D-square and Smith's mean measure of divergence (MMDs), make it possible to describe overall patterns of variation and interpret results in light of population history. However, these classic statistical procedures do not necessarily address population structure (Relethford, 1991, 1996). The estimation of specific parameters relevant to population structure such as population dynamics, gene flow, and genetic drift based on phenotypic data was not attempted until Relethford and Blangero's (1990) R-matrix method, originally used with allele frequency data, was applied to craniometric data (Relethford and Hapending, 1990; Relethford, 1994, 1996, 2002, 2004; Relethford and Harpending, 1994; Powell and Neves, 1999; Steadman, 2001; González-José et al., 2003, 2005; Roseman and Weaver, 2004; Stojanowski, 2004; Sardi et al., 2005; Schilacii and Stojanowski, 2005; Scherer, 2007). However, it requires metric data.

It is generally accepted that nonmetric cranial (and dental) traits are under moderate to high genetic control, selectively more neutral than metric traits, and useful for investigating population history and microevolutionary events (Ossenberg, 1986, 2002; Hauser and Stefano, 1989; Hanihara et al., 2003). However, R-matrix application to nonmetric morphological traits is not yet widely performed (Leigh et al., 2004; Pilbow, 2006; Hanihara, 2008). At the very least, no qualitative morphological studies explicitly considered the potential effect of gene flow, genetic drift, and population size on among-group variation within a relatively small geographic region.

Given these background, the purpose of the present study is to extend the R-matrix approach developed for quantitative morphological data to qualitative phenotypic (nonmetric) data for considering the potential effects of gene flow and genetic drift on the patterns of among-population variation of the Ainu using the data of effective population size.

MATERIALS AND METHODS

In the present study, morphological variation in 24 nonmetric cranial traits was examined. The cranial materials of the Ainu are derived from two major geographic regions: Hokkaido and Sakhalin Island. The cranial series of the Hokkaido Ainu are divided into seven local groups. The boundaries of these local groups are identical to the administrative divisions, which correspond almost exactly to the watersheds (Hanihara et al., 2008). The information on the Ainu groups and the three comparative series is given in Table 1. Figure 1 illustrates the location of the samples used. The nonmetric cranial traits used for assessing phenotypic variation and biological distance were listed in Table 2.

Table 1. Material used and the brief information

Sample Name	Brief Information
Recent Ainu	
Sakhalin Island	Sakaehama, Honto villages, Sakhalin Island (Kyoto Univ)
Hokkaido	
Northeast	
Soya	Esashi, Wakkanai, Rebun Island (Univ. of Tokyo, Sapporo Medical Univ.)
Abashiri	Abashiri, Monbetsu, Shari, and Toro (Univ. of Tokyo, Sapporo Medical Univ.)
Nemuro	Nemuro (Univ. of Tokyo, Sapporo Medical Univ.)
Central	
Tokachi	Hiroo and Ohtsu(Utsunai) (Univ. of Tokyo)
Hidaka	Urakawa, Atsubetsu, Horoizumi, Mitsuishi, Saru, Shizunai, and Urakawa regions (Univ. of Tokyo, Sapporo Medical Univ.)
Western	
Ishikari	Sapporo and the neighboring city (Univ. of Tokyo, Sapporo Medical Univ.)
Shiribeshi	Otaru, Yoichi, and Iwanai (Univ. of Tokyo)
Comparative samples	
Jomon/Hokkaido and Tohoku	Usu-Moshiri, Kitakogane, Takasago, Irie (Abuta) Shell mounds; Motowa-Nish (Muroran), Yakumo-Kotan (Oshima), Tenneru (Kushiro) Shimamaki (Shiribeshi) and other sites in Hokkaido Ebishima, Nakazawahama, Ohora, Hosoura (Iwate Prefecture); Sanganji (Fukushima Prefecture); Sakai-Numazu, Hashimotogakoi, Satohama (Miyagi Prefecture); Kashidokoro (Akita Prefecture) and Other sites: From Tohoku region of Eastern Japan (Univ. of Tokyo, National Museum of Nature and Science)
Okhotsk culture people	5-12 century A.D. Hamanaka, Rebun Island; Ohmisaki, Soya; Moyoro, Abashiri; Susuya, Sakhalin (Hokkaido Univ, Sapporo Medical Univ., Kyoto Univ.)
Modern Japanese	Mainly from Tokyo (Univ. of Tokyo)

The R-matrix method developed by Relethford and Blangero (1990) was applied to estimating regional variation in qualitative phenotypic traits. Computation of R-matrix requires certain quantities such as deviation and covariance matrices, Fst, etc., weighted by population size. For weighting, the census population sizes of the Ainu in 1875 are adopted (Hanihara et al., 2008), since the Ainu materials used in this study consist largely of those collected by Y. Koganei in the late 19th century (Koganei, 1893). The sample sizes and the census population sizes of the Ainu are shown in Table 3. To conduct R-matrix method, moreover, an estimate of average heritability for nonmetric cranial traits used is required. In this study, average heritability values of 0.50 for nonmetric cranial traits were used. The appropriateness of the estimates of the average heritability of $h^2 = 0.50$, moderate estimate for genetic contribution, is indicated by several researches based on family study and on the relationship between unilateral and bilateral expression of bilateral traits (Lane, 1978; Ossenberg, 1981; Sjøvold, 1984; Hauser and Stefano, 1989).

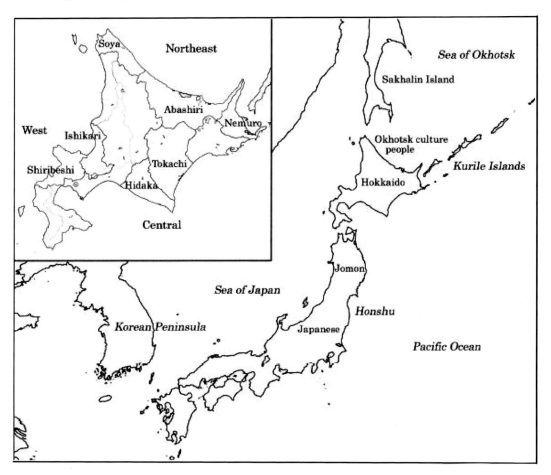

Figure 1. Geographical location of the cranial samples used in the present study.

The scoring procedures for each trait are further described in Hanihara and Ishida (2001a-e). All traits were dichotomized into categories of present or absent. The previous study showed that in many traits: (1) the frequency distributions by sex were not significantly different; and (2) the intertrait correlation between every pair of traits and the right and left side difference in bilateral trait estimated by χ^2 and Fisher's exact probability tests are not significant. Based on these findings, I have selected the individual count method (if a trait was present on either or both side, it was scored as present in bilateral trait), and to use the sex-combined dataset.

Table 2. The 24 nonmetric cranial traits used and references

Traits	References
1. Medial palatine canal	Dodo (1974), Hanihara and Ishida (2001d)
2. Hypoglossal canal bridging	Dodo (1974, 1987)
3. Condylar canal patent	Dodo (1974), Hauser and Stefano (1989)
4. Tympanic dehiscence	Dodo (1974), Hanihara and Ishida (2001c)
5. Foramen of Vesalius	Dodo (1974), Hauser and Stefano (1989)
6. Precondylar tubercle	Hanihara and Ishida (2001d)
7. Paracondylar process	Dodo (1974), Hauser and Stefano (1989)
8. Condylus tertius	Hanihara and Ishida (2001d)
9. Jugular foramen bridging	Dodo (1986a, 1986b)
10. Ovale-spinosum confluence	Dodo (1974), Hanihara and Ishida (2001c)
11. Pterygo-spinous foramen	Dodo (1974, 1987)
12. Supraorbital foramen	Dodo (1974, 1987)
13. Accessory infraorbital foramen	Haninara and Ishida (2001e)
14. Metopism	Haninara and Ishida (2001c)
15. Transverse zygomatic suture vestige	
16. Ossicle at the lambda	Dodo (1974), Hanihara and Ishida (2001b)
17. Inca bone	Hanihara and Ishida (2001a)
18. Parietal notch bone	Dodo (1974), Hanihara and Ishida (2001b)
19. Asterionic bone	Dodo (1974), Hanihara and Ishida (2001b)
20. Biasterionic suture	Dodo (1974), Hanihara and Ishida (2001c)
21. Mylohyoid bridging	Dodo (1974), Jidoi et al. (2000)
22. Accessory mental foramen	Hanihara and Ishida (2001e)
23. Lambdoid bone	Hauser and Stefano (1989)
24. Occipitomastoid bone	Dodo (1974), Hanihara and Ishida (2001b)

Table 3. Number of samples and census sizes of the local Ainu populations

	N	Population size at 1875
Recent Ainu		
Sakhalin Island	46	2,372
Hokkaido		
Soya	15	358
Abashiri	20	951
Nemuro	14	472
Tokachi	29	1,475
Hidaka	67	5,236
Ishikari	16	3,868
Shiribeshi	25	799
Camparative samples		
Jomon/Hokkaido-Tohoku	115	-
Okhotsk people	33	-
Modern Japanese	57	-

It is generally accepted that the nonmetric skeletal variants can be regarded as threshold characters, following the model proposed by Falconer (1967). The model assumes that the trait liability is normally distributed, and can be broken by the imposition of a threshold into presence/absence states (summarized by Hauser and Stefano, 1989). Assuming an underlying multivariate normal distribution of the liabilities, Blangero and Williams-Blangero (1991, 1993) estimated the values of liabilities and the variance-covariance matrices using marginal maximum likelihood method and Monte Carlo maximum likelihood approach. Konigsberg (1990) and Konigsberg et al. (1993) estimated the thresholds and the variance-covariance matrices using probit regression analysis and maximum likelihood method, respectively. With recent theoretical developments from Bayesian statistics, the Gibbs sampler, a Markov Chain Monte Carlo (MCMC) method was used to estimate liabilities for the numerical evaluation of high dimensional multivariate normal integrals and for the use of Fst statistic (Leigh and Konigsberg, 1996; Leigh et al., 2004).

In the present study, application of R-matrix method was extended to nonmetric cranial data using a pooled within-group variance-covariance matrix estimated with maximum likelihood method (tetrachoric correlation matrix) and standard deviation units derived from threshold values for each trait.

Tetrachoric correlation matrix estimated with maximum likelihood method is an extension of Relethford and Blangero's (1990) pooled within-group variance-covariance matrix calculated from standardized metric data to cover nonmetric traits caused by thresholds on polygenically determined liabilities (Blangero and Williams-Blangero, 1991; Konigsberg et al., 1993). The tetrachoric correlation is appropriate for binary nonmetric morphological data which reflect an underlying normal distribution of some determining factor (Hallgrímsson et al., 2004). The codivergence matrix $\mathbf{C}$ is computed as

$$\mathbf{C} = \Delta\, \mathbf{G}^{-1}\, \Delta',$$

where $\mathbf{G}$ is a matrix of pooled within group additive genetic variance- covariance matrix between traits calculated from tetrachoric correlation matrix, Δ is a g by t matrix consisting of deviation of group means of the thresholds from the total means pooled over all populations weighted by population size, and the prime (') indicates matrix transposition (g; number of groups, and t; number of traits). Within group tetrachoric correlation matrix is averaged over all populations weighted by population size. The thresholds for the Δ were estimated using the univariate probit analysis as follows:

$$P\,(t = 1) = \Phi[f\,(x)],$$

where $P\,(t = 1)$ is the probability that an individual will display a particular discrete trait, $\Phi[f\,(x)]$ is the standardized normal integral from negative infinity to $f\,(x)$ (Konigsberg et al., 1993).

Calculation of the G-matrix from tetrachoric correlation matrix (T-matrix) requires an estimate of average heritability for nonmetric dental traits. Using average heritability of the traits (h^2), G-matrix is calculated as

$$\mathbf{G} = h^2\, \mathbf{T}.$$

The C-matrix is finally divided by t to give an average value over all traits. The distinction of this procedure is made clear in the appendix in Relethford et al. (1997). The Fst, the ratio of among-group variation to total variation, is defined as

$$Fst = (\sum w_i C_{ii}) / (2t + \sum w_i C_{ii})$$

where w_i is the weighting factor, the relative size of population i, defined as

$$w_i = Ni / \Sigma Nj,$$

and where Nj is the effective size of population j (Relethford and Blangero, 1990; Relethford, 1994; Relethford and Harpending, 1994). Using C-matrix and Fst value obtained, the R-matrix is computed as

$$\mathbf{R} = \mathbf{C} \, (1 - Fst) / 2t.$$

The diagonal elements of the R-matrix represent the genetic distances of each population to the "centroid" defined in terms of the average trait frequencies over all populations (Relethford and Blangero, 1990; Relthford and Harpending, 1994). Under an equilibrium between gene flow and genetic drift, intra-group variation and distance from the centroid, defined as r_{ii}, are expected to be related in a linear fashion (Relethford and Harpending, 1994). Relethford and Harpending (1994) modified this model for use with quantitative traits as

$$E[\bar{v}_i] = \bar{v}_w \, (1 - r_{ii}) / (1 - Fst).$$

The expected average phenotypic variation in group i ($E[\bar{v}_i]$) is a function of the pooled average within-group phenotypic variation over all groups ($\bar{v}_w$), the distance from the centroid defined by r_{ii}, and intergroup variation presented by Fst. In the present study, within-group phenotypic variation in each trait is estimated using the method of bootstrap resampling of the original data in each group with 500 replications (Shao and Tu, 1995; Manly, 1997).

Biological distances between every pair of the samples were transformed from R-matrix as follows (Relethford and Harpending, 1994),

$$d_{ij}^{\,2} = r_{ii} + r_{jj} - 2r_{ij.}$$

The pattern of morphological affinities between recent Ainu groups and the neighboring populations was analyzed by applying Torgerson's (1952) metric multidimensional scaling method to the distance matrix obtained.

RESULTS

The frequencies of occurrence for all 24 traits in the 11 samples are listed in Table 4. As often happens with archaeologically derived remains, small sample size is a factor restricting multivariate analytical approaches. The threshold model for discrete traits is more effective in analyzing population affinities than classic frequency based model such as MMDs when sample size is not enough large (Konigsberg, 1990; Konigsberg et al., 1993; Bedrick et al., 2000; Irish, 2006). As Irish (2006) emphasizes, a tetrachoric correlation matrix used here is calculated within each sample and pooled using sample size for each trait pair, producing weighted average correlations.

The observed, expected, and residual variance together with the average dispersion of the samples around the centroid, r_{ii}, calculated using average heritabilities of the 24 nonmetric cranial traits of $h^2 = 0.50$ for the eight local samples of the Ainu are given in Table 5. Figure 2 illustrates the plot of observed variance versus genetic distance from the centroid (r_{ii}) with the expected regression line based on the expected variance shown in Table 5. The Nemuro, Soya, and to a lesser extent Ishikari samples show greater phenotypic variation than expected, suggesting gene flow from outside the region. On the other hand, the Hidaka and Sakhalin samples are plotted under the expected regression line, suggesting isolation and/or genetic drift.

To avoid a potential influence of nonrandom sampling effects caused by small sample sizes that may artificially bias regional variations, the seven local Hokkaido Ainu series were grouped into three regional clusters, northeastern, central, and western groups (Table 1). The northeastern Ainu sample consists of three local groups, Soya, Abashiri, and Nemuro, that overlap the area containing the sites of the Okhotsk culture which have been discovered thus far (Figure 1). The results of the analysis using combined datasets are presented in Table 6 and Figure 3. Both the western and northeastern Hokkaido Ainu are positive outliers to the expected regression line, as expected in the previous analysis shown in Figure 2. The difference between the two results, such as the changing position of the Sakhalin Ainu, is likely a function of the relative distance from the population centroid represented by r_{ii}.

Relethford (1991) regarded the relationship between r_{ii}, the within-group elements of the R-matrix, and the reciprocal of census population size ($1/N_i$) as a rough measure of the overall potential for genetic drift/gene flow. The r_{ii} values, the genetic distances to the population centroid, are expected to increase as a consequence of genetic drift and decrease as a result of admixture in a closed system or kin-structured migration (Relethford, 1991; Relethford and Harpending, 1994). In Figure 4a and 4b, the r_{ii} are plotted against the reciprocal of census population size for the eight local groups and the four regional groups, respectively. A plot of the samples shows roughly linear, suggesting the positive association between r_{ii} and $1/N_i$ expected under a situation of genetic drift (Relethford, 1991). The scattergrams show that the samples from western Hokkaido, the Ishikari and Shiribeshi groups, and the Sakhalin Ainu sample have larger r_{ii} values than expected on the basis of population size. In Figure 4b, moreover, the sample of northeastern group has more or less smaller r_{ii} values than expected.

Table 4. Frequencies of 24 nonmetric cranial traits in the 11 cranial series from Ainu and neighboring populations

	Ainu/Sakhalin		Ainu/Soya		Ainu/Abashiri		Ainu/Nemuro		Ainu/Tokachi		Ainu/Hidaka		Ainu/Ishikari		Ainu/Shiribeshi	
	p	N	p	N	p	N	p	N	p	N	p	N	p	N	p	N
Medial palatine canal	2.63	38	30.77	13	17.65	17	0.04*	7	20	20	15.38	52	40	15	40.91	22
Hypoglossal canal bridging	45.45	44	28.57	14	50	18	15.38	13	40.74	27	38.71	62	31.25	16	50	24
Condylar canal patent	92.5	40	85.71	14	94.74	19	84.62	13	84.62	26	93.33	60	86.67	15	91.3	23
Tympanic dehiscence	25	44	7.14	14	21.05	19	30.77	13	11.11	27	30.16	63	0.02*	16	21.74	23
Foramen of Vesalius	30.23	43	15.38	13	26.32	19	18.18	11	32	25	22.03	59	25	16	13.64	22
Precondylar tubercle	12.82	39	7.69	13	5.88	17	0.02*	12	16.67	24	1.75	57	18.75	16	0.01*	24
Paracondylar process	16.67	30	10	10	12.5	16	16.67	6	20	20	24.32	37	30.77	13	18.75	16
Condylus tertius	0.01*	41	0.02*	14	0.01*	18	0.02*	13	0.01*	26	5.26	19	6.25	16	4.17	24
Jugular foramen bridging	23.81	42	23.08	13	11.11	18	15.38	13	20	25	15.25	59	25	16	21.74	23
Ovale-spinosum confluence	2.44	41	0.02*	14	15.79	19	0.03*	10	7.69	26	6.78	59	25	16	4.35	23
Pterygo-spinous foramen	4.88	41	7.69	13	0.01*	19	0.03*	10	15.38	26	4.55	44	6.67	15	8.7	23
Supraorbital foramen	55.81	43	33.33	15	33.33	18	21.43	14	19.23	26	20.34	59	31.25	16	27.27	22
Accessory infraorbital foramen	22.22	36	18.18	11	22.22	18	33.33	6	10	20	21.05	19	13.33	15	0.01*	22
Metopism	0.01*	45	6.67	15	0.01*	20	0.02		14	0.01*	28	4.62		65	0.02*	16
Transverse zygomatic suture vestige	7.41	27	80	10	33.33	15	33.33	3	28.57	14	17.24	29	11.76	12	11.76	17
Ossicle at the lambda	0.01*	43	0.02*	15	0.01*	18	0.02*	14	0.01*	28	1.59	63	0.02*	15	0.01*	24
Inca bone	0.01*	44	0.02*	15	5.26	19	0.02*	13	0.01*	28	3.08	65	0.02*	16	4.35	23
Parietal notch bone	18.18	44	21.43	14	11.11	18	23.08	13	15.38	26	8.47	59	6.67	15	13.64	22
Asterionic bone	6.82	44	14.29	14	5.56	18	0.02*	13	7.41	27	6.78	59	18.75	16	36.36	22
Biasterionic suture	11.63	43	6.67	15	44.44	18	30.77	13	10.71	28	15.87	63	25	16	18.18	22

	Ainu/Sakhalin		Ainu/Soya		Ainu/Abashiri		Ainu/Nemuro		Ainu/Tokachi		Ainu/Hidaka		Ainu/Ishikari		Ainu/Shiribeshi	
	p	N	p	N	p	N	p	N	p	N	p	N	p	N	p	N
Mylohyoid bridging	14.29	35	12.5	8	20	15	9.09	11	25	12	22.64	53	7.69	13	14.29	14
Accessory mental foramen	17.95	39	25	8	25	16	16.67	12	50	12	15.69	51	30.77	13	7.14	14
Foramen of Vesalius	30.23	43	15.38	13	26.32	19	18.18	11	32	25	22.03	59	25	16	13.64	22
Lambdoid bone	27.91	43	66.67	15	57.89	19	38.46	13	21.43	28	49.18	61	25	16	52.38	21
Occipitomastooid bone	9.3	43	28.57	14	27.78	18	38.46	13	14.81	27	15.52	58	0.02*	16	13.04	23

*, The frequency p = 0 is replaced by p = 1/4n (Bartlett's adjustment)

Table 4. (continued)

	Jomon		Okhotsk		Japan	
	p	N	p	N	p	N
Medial palatine canal	23.81	42	5.88	17	12.28	57
Hypoglossal canal bridging	25.58	43	21.05	19	21.05	57
Condylar canal patent	88.24	17	93.75	16	82.14	56
Tympanic dehiscence	18.57	70	29.63	27	43.86	57
Foramen of Vesalius	33.33	30	40	15	32.14	56
Precondylar tubercle	2.33	43	5.88	17	1.75	57
Paracondylar process	50	18	50	10	21.43	56
Condylus tertius	0.01*	34	0.02*	12	1.79	56
Jugular foramen bridging	0.01*	18	10	20	23.21	56
Ovale-spinosum confluence	0.01*	30	0.02*	15	1.75	57
Pterygo-spinous foramen	0.01*	17	0.02*	12	1.75	57
Supraorbital foramen	10.98	82	44.44	27	49.12	57
Accessory infraorbital foramen	13.33	15	21.34	14	14.29	56
Metopism	10.1	99	0.01*	29	5.26	57
Transverse zygomatic suture vestige	45.16	31	7.69	13	3.57	56
Ossicle at the lambda	4.94	81	0.01*	26	1.79	56
Inca bone	1.15	87	3.7	27	1.75	57
Parietal notch bone	25	32	31.58	19	21.43	56
Asterionic bone	8.33	48	5.88	17	5.36	56
Biasterionic suture	39.58	48	21.74	23	12.73	55
Mylohyoid bridging	28.07	57	13.33	15	3.77	53
Accessory mental foramen	19.23	78	23.53	17	12.96	54
Foramen of Vesalius	33.33	30	40	15	32.14	56
Lambdoid bone	71.43	35	77.78	18	33.96	53
Occipitomastooid bone	10.53	38	31.25	16	16.36	55

*, The frequency p = 0 is replaced by p = 1/4n (Bartlett's adjustment)

Table 5. Eight local samples of the Ainu: genetic distance to the centroid (r_{ii}), observed, expected, and residual variances computed using an average heritability of $h^2 = 0.50$

Sample name	r_{ii}	Observed	Expected Variance	Residual Variance	S.E. Variance
Sakhalin Ainu	0.1403	0.0027	0.0067	-0.0041	0.0000
Ainu/Soya	0.2358	0.0094	0.0060	0.0034	0.0000
Ainu/Abashiri	0.1142	0.0071	0.0069	0.0001	0.0000
Ainu/Nemuro	0.1933	0.0123	0.0063	0.0060	0.0003
Ainu/Tokachi	0.0966	0.0059	0.0071	-0.0011	0.0000
Ainu/Hidaka	0.0526	0.0025	0.0074	-0.0049	0.0000
Ainu/Ishikari	0.1503	0.0082	0.0067	0.0015	0.0000
Ainu/Shiribeshi	0.1863	0.0055	0.0064	-0.0009	0.0000

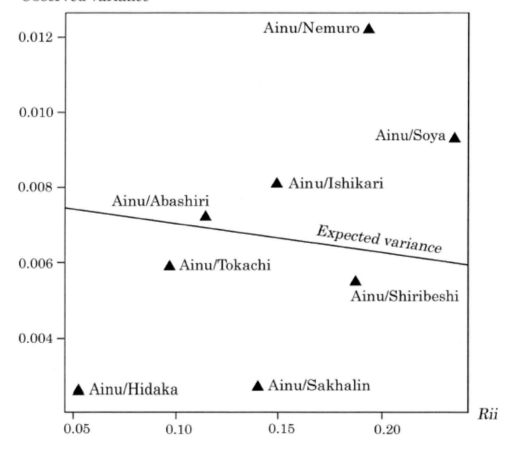

Figure 2. Plot of observed phenotypic variance versus genetic distance from the centroid (r_{ii}) for the eight local Ainu samples. The line indicates the expected regression line derived from Relethford and Blangero's (1990) model.

Table 6. Four regional samples of the Ainu: genetic distance to the centroid (r_{ii}), observed, expected, and residual variances computed using an average heritability of $h^2 = 0.50$

Sample name	r_{ii}	Observed	Expected Variance	Residual Variance	S.E. Variance
Sakhalin Ainu	0.1416	0.0027	0.0025	0.0003	0.0000
Ainu/Northeast	0.0972	0.0030	0.0026	0.0004	0.0000
Ainu/Central	0.0144	0.0016	0.0029	-0.0012	0.0000
Ainu/Western	0.0661	0.0033	0.0027	0.0006	0.0000

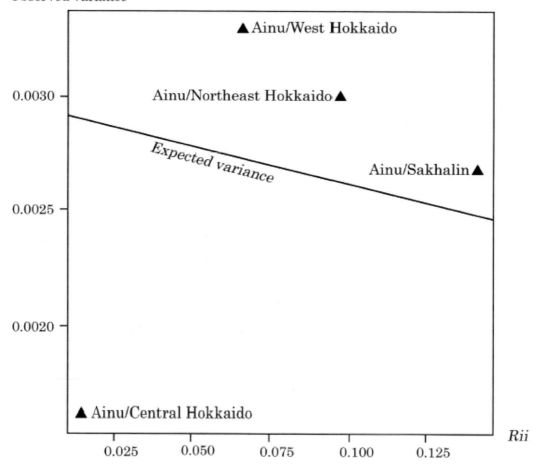

Figure 3. Plot of observed phenotypic variance versus genetic distance from the centroid (r_{ii}) for the four regional Ainu samples. The line indicates the expected regression line.

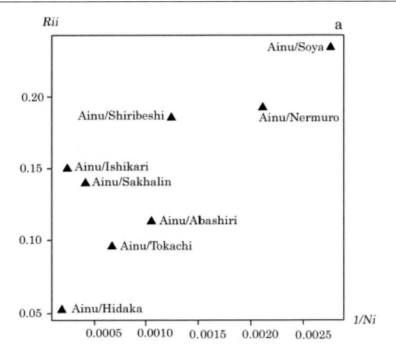

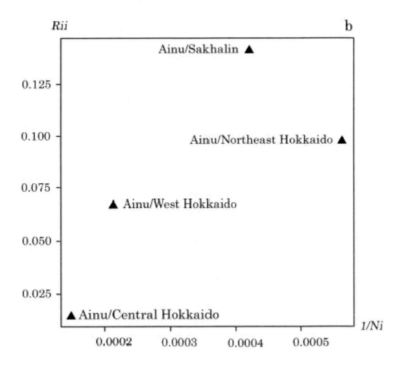

Figure 4. Scattergram of distance from the centroid (r_{ii}) based on nonmetric cranial data versus the reciprocal of census population size of the Ainu in 1875, for the eight local Ainu samples (a) and the four regional Ainu samples (b).

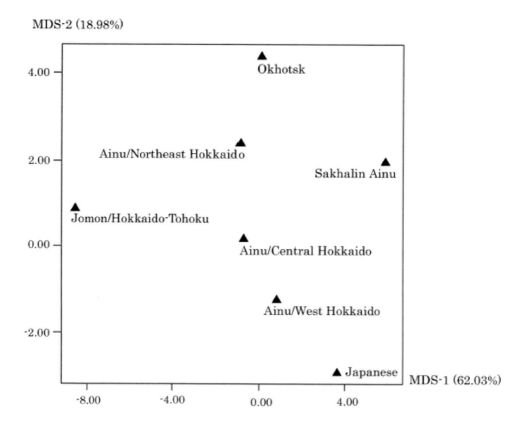

Figure 5. Two dimensional scattergram drawn by multidimensional scaling, based on the distance matrix transformed from R-matrix.

Given the estimates of the differential gene flow from outside sources and genetic drift, possible patterns of migration and admixture are examined using three comparative series (Table 1). The two dimensional expression of the intergroup relationship that results from multidimensional scaling applied to the distance matrix converted from R-matrix is shown in Figure 5. Using the first two dimensions, 81% of the total variance is expressed. The most peripherally positioned samples are the Jomon, Okhotsk culture people, and recent Japanese. The four Ainu series fall within the constellation of the three comparative samples. The western Ainu sample is closest to the Japanese sample. The northeastern Hokkaido Ainu is closest to the Okhotsk Culture sample, followed by the Sakhalin Ainu sample. The findings suggest the possible genetic influence of the Okhotsk culture people to the northeastern Hokkaido Ainu on the one hand, and of the non-Ainu Japanese to the western Hokkaido Ainu on the other hand.

DISCUSSION

Several recent studies for the origin and affinities of the Ainu have suggested the effects of gene flow from Northeast Asian continent during the post-Jomon periods (Shigematsu et al., 2002; Sato et al., 2005, 2009; Adachi et al., 2009). This paper extends previous craniometric studies showing the influence of migration from outside source and admixture on phenotypic structure in the local groups of the Hokkaido Ainu (Hanihara et al., 2008). The present qualitative morphological analyses generate essentially convergent results obtained by craniometric analyses (Hanihara et al., 2008).

A possible genetic influence from external source to at least the Ainu from the coastal region along the Sea of Okhotsk and the easternmost region of Hokkaido are suggested from observed- and expected-variance comparison. Likewise, the Ainu from western part of Hokkaido shows positive deviation from the expected variation, explicable by gene flow from outside source and admixture.

As shown in Figure 5, moreover, the Ainu series from the coastal region of the Sea of Okhotsk are more northern-like than are the other Ainu series on the one hand, and the western Hokkaido Ainu groups are more southern-like on the other hand. Such findings suggest possible admixture between the Okhotsk culture people and northeastern Hokkaido inhabitants during 5-12th century A.D., and between recent non-Ainu Japanese from main-island Japan, Honshu, and western Hokkaido Ainu as indicated previously (Yamaguchi, 1982; Sato et al., 2007; Adachi et al., 2009; Hanihara et al., 2008).

For the western and northeastern Ainu groups, however, the r_{ii} and $1/N_i$ relationship analysis shown in Figure 4 provides different results obtained by variance analysis presented in Figures 2 and 3. The results suggest possible effect of genetic drift on the western groups and gene flow on northeastern groups. According to Relethford (1991), the use of a potential genetic drift/admixture analyses makes certain assumptions that must be paid attention: 1) all census population sizes are assumed to be equally proportional to effective population sizes; 2) all populations treated have the same time depth since founding; and 3) the population sizes have remained constant over time. The first assumption requires that age structure and other factors influencing the effective population size should be distributed randomly through the region of analysis. However, this assumption is common to many models of population structure but cannot be tested precisely (Relethford, 1991). The second assumption may not critical because the present cranial series of the Ainu are descendants of the prehistoric Jomon people in Japan (Howells, 1986; Brace and Hunt, 1990; Dodo and Ishida, 1990; Dodo and Kawakubo, 2002). Regarding the third assumption, the use of a single census year's figures to infer past drift and/or admixture effects is valid only to the extent that population sizes have not changed dramatically (Relethford, 1991). Long-term effects of population growth or decline may affect on the results shown in Figures 3 and 4 (Rogers and Harpending, 1986; Relethford, 1991). More importantly, admixture between morphologically and genetically distinguishable populations may increase not only the variations but also the r_{ii} value representing the genetic distance to the population centroid (Relethford and Blangero, 1990; Relethford, 1991; Relethford and Harpending, 1994).

It is well known that the morphological features of recent Ainu are quite different from those of modern Japanese (Turner, 1987, 1990; Brace and Hunt, 1990; Hanihara, 1991; Dodo and Ishida, 1990; Hanihara et al., 1998, 2008). A possible external source of heterogeneous genes brought by non-Ainu Japanese may be a cause for larger r_{ii} value than expected on the basis of population size in western part of Hokkaido (shown in Figure 4).

The island of Hokkaido was not fully incorporated into the Japanese homeland until towards the end of the 19th century. From the early 17th century, there had been small Japanese settlements around the castle town of Matsumae in the extreme southwest of the island, but little attempt was made to push further north or east except by small bands of loggers and fishermen. Following the Meiji Restoration in the 19th century, the city of Sapporo in the central of Ishikari subprefecture was laid out as the seat of Hokkaido's colonial administration. Many of settlers in 1800s emigrated to Sapporo and its vicinity, southwestern part of Hokkaido. A possible genetic impact of non-Ainu Japanese on southwestern Hokkaido Ainu suggested by this study agree with such pioneering history of Hokkaido.

Ishida (1999) and Komesu et al. (2008) demonstrated that the Ainu and the Okhotsk culture people share to some degree similar characteristics for nonmetric cranial traits, which can be traced back to those of the Neolithic Jomon and Northeast Asians. At the very least, the Ainu is more closely related to the Okhotsk culture people than to non-Ainu Japanese (Ishida, 1995, 1996, 1999). This may allow us to acknowledge the different results between observed- and expected-variance analysis and $r_{ii} - 1/N_i$ relationship analysis for western and northeastern Hokkaido Ainu groups.

Classic distance analyses such as Smith's MMD distance for nonmetric data can describe overall patterns of variation and interpopulation similarities (Relethford, 1991, 1996; Relethford and Harpending, 1994). However, many factors such as gene flow, genetic drift, climatic and subsistence adaptation, etc., which have had an impact on morphological variation and affinities between populations, tend be erased or even obscured in the final output presented by scattergrams and/or tree diagrams (Relethford, 1991, 1996). The present extension of R-matrix approach to nonmetric cranial data provides results that are consistent with not only recent genetic and craniometric evidence but also archaeological and prehistoric knowledge for waves of migrants from the neighboring regions into Hokkaido (Amano, 2003; Tajima et al., 2004; Sato et al., 2007; Hanihara et al., 2008).

ACKNOWLEDGMENTS

I wish to express my sincere thanks to T. Amano of Hokkaido University Museum, Sapporo; M. Matsumura of the Department of Anatomy, Sapporo Medical University, Sapporo; Y. Dodo of the Department of Anatomy, Tohoku University School of Medicine, Sendai; G. Suwa of the Department of Anthropology, University Museum, The University of Tokyo, Tokyo; H. Baba and Y. Mizoguchi of the Department of Anthropology, National Museum of Nature and Science, Tokyo; K. Katayama of the Department of Zoology, Kyoto University, Kyoto; for their kind permission to study the materials under their care.

REFERENCES

Adachi N, Shinoda K, Umetsu K, Matsumura H. 2009. Mitochondrial DNA analysis of Jomon skeletons from the Funadomari site, Hokkaido, and its implication for the origin of Native Americans. *Am J Phys Anthropol.* DOI: 10.1002/ajpa20923.

Bedrick EJ, Lapidus J, Powell JF. 2000. Estimating the Mahalanobis distance from mixed continuous and discrete data. *Biometrics,* 56:394-401.

Betti L, Balloux F, Amos W, Hanihara T, Manica A. 2009. Distance from Africa, not climate, explains within-population phenotypic diversity in humans. *Proc R Soc B*: doi:10.1098/rspb.2008.1563.

Blangero J, Williams-Blangero S. 1991. Estimating biological distance from dichotomous threshold traits. *Am J Phys Anthropol Suppl.* 12:51-52.

Blangero J, Williams-Blangero S. 1993. A quantitative genetic method for calculating genetic distances from dermatoglyphic pattern types. *Am J Phys Anthropol Suppl.* 16:57-58.

Brace CL, Hunt KD. 1990. A nonracial craniofacial perspective on human variation A(ustralia) to Z(uni). *Am J Phys Anthropol.* 82:341-360.

Cavalli-Sforza LL, Menozzi P, Piazza A. 1994. The history and geography of human genes. Princeton: Princeton University Press.

Dodo Y, Ishida H. 1990. Population history of Japan as viewed from cranial nonmetric variation. *J Anthropol Soc Nippon.* 98:269-287.

Dodo Y, Kawakubo Y. 2002. Cranial affinities of the Epi-Jomon inhabitants in Hokkaido, Japan. *Anthropol Sci.* 110:1-32.

Eller E 1999. Population substructure and isolation by distance in three continental regions. *Am J Phys Anthropol.* 108:147-15.

Falconer DS. 1967. The inheritance of liability to disease with variable age of onset, with particular reference to diabetes mellitus. *Ann Hum Genet.* 31:1-20.

Fix AG. 1978. The role of kin-structured migration in genetic microdifferentiation. *Ann Hum Genet.* 41:329-339.

González-José R, González-Martin A, Hernández M, Pucciarelli HM, Sardi M, Rosales A, Molen SV. 2003. Craniometric evidence for Palaeoamerican survival in Baja California. *Nature*, 425:62-65.

González-José R, Neves W, Lahr MM, González S, Pucciarelli H, Martínez MH, Correal G. 2005. Late Pleistocene/Holocene craniofacial morphology in Mesoamerican Paleoindians: implications for the peopling of the New World. *Am J Phys Anthropol.* 128:772-780.

Hallgrímsson B, Donnabháin ÓB, Walters GB, Cooper DML, Guðbjartsson D, Stefánsson K. 2004. Composition of the founding population of Iceland: biological distance and morphological variation in early historic Atlantic Europe. *Am J Phys Anthropol.* 124:257-274.

Hammer MF, Horai S. 1995. Y chromosomal DNA variation and the peopling of Japan. *Am J Hum Genet.* 46:115-125.

Hanihara K. 1991. Dual structure model for the population history of the Japanese. *Japan Rev.* 2:1-33.

Hanihara T. 2008. Morphological variation of major human populations based on nonmetric dental traits. *Am J Phys Anthropol.* 136:169-182.

Hanihara T, Ishida H. 2009. Regional differences in craniofacial diversity and the population history of Jomon Japan. *Am J Phys Anthropol.* DOI 10.1002/ajpa.20985.

Hanihara T, Ishida H, Dodo Y. 1998. Place of the Hokkaido Ainu (northern Japan) among circumpolar and other peoples of the world: a comparison of the frequency variation of discrete cranial traits. *Internatl J Circumpolar Health,* 57:257-275.

Hanihara T, Ishida H. 2001. Os incae: variation in frequency in major human population groups. *J Anat.* 198:137-152.

Hanihara T, Ishida H. 2001. Frequency variations of discrete cranial traits in major human populations. I. Supernumerary ossicle variations. *J Anat.* 198:689-706.

Hanihara T, Ishida H. 2001. Frequency variations of discrete cranial traits in major human populations. II. Hypostotic variations. *J Anat.* 198:707-725.

Hanihara T, Ishida H. 2001. Frequency variations of discrete cranial traits in major human populations. III. Hyperostotic variations. *J Anat.* 199:251-272.

Hanihara T, Ishida H. 2001. Frequency variations of discrete cranial traits in major human populations. IV. Vessel and nerve related variations. *J Anat.* 199:273-287.

Hanihara T, Yoshida M, Ishida H. 2008. Craniometric variation of the Ainu: an assessment of differential gene flow from Northeast Asia to northern Japan, Hokkaido. *Am J Phys Anthropol.* 137:283-293.

Harpending H, Rogers A. 2000. Genetic perspectives of human origins and differentiation. *Annu Rev Genomics Hum Genet.* 1:361-85.

Hauser GV, De Stefano GFR. 1989. Epigenetic variants of the human skull. Stuttgart: Schweizerbart.

Horai S, Murayama K, Hayasaka K, Matsubayashi S, Hattori Y, Fucharoen G, Harihara S, Park KS, Omoto K, Pan IH. 1996. mtDNA polymorphism in East Asian populations, with special reference to the peopling of Japan. *Am J Hum Genet,* 59:579-590.

Howells WW. 1986. Physical anthropology of the prehistoric Japanese. In: Pearson RJ, editor. Windows on the Japanese past: studies in archaeology and prehistory. Ann Arbor: Center for Japanese Studies, The University of Michigan. p 85-99.

Hudson MJ. 2004. The perverse realities of change: world system incorporation and the Okhotsk culture of Hokkaido. *J Anthropol Archaeol.* 23:290-308.

Irish JD. 2006. Who were the ancient Egyptians? Dental affinities among Neolithic through postdynastic peoples. *Am J Phys Anthropol.* 129:529-543.

Ishida H. 1994. Skeletal morphology of the Okhotsk people on Sakhalin Island. *Anthropol Sci.* 102:257-269.

Ishida H. 1995. Nonmetric cranial variation of Northeast Asian populations and their population affinities. *Anthropol Sci.* 103:385-401.

Ishida H. 1996. Metric and nonmetric cranial variation of the prehistoric Okhotsk people. *Anthropol Sci.* 104:233-258.

Ishida H. 1999. Ancient people of the North Pacific rim: Ainu biological relationships with their neighbors. In: Fitzhugh WW, Dubreuil CO, editors. Ainu: spirit of a northern people. Washington DC: National Museum of Natural History. p 52-56.

Jorde LB, Rogers AR, Bamshad M, Watkins WS, Krakowiak PA, Sung S, Kere J, Harpending HC. 1997. Microsatellite diversity and the demographic history of modern humans. *Proc Natl Acad Sci USA,* 94:3100-3103.

Koganei Y. 1893. Beiträge zur physischen Anthropologie der Ainu. I. Untersuchungen am Skelet. Mittheilungen aus der medicinischen Facultät der Kaiserlich-Japanischen Universität 2:1-249.

Komesu A, Hanihara T, Amano T, Ono H, Yoneda M, Dodo Y, Fukumine T, Ishida H. 2008. Nonmetric cranial variation in human skeletal remains associated with Okhotsk culture. *Anthropol Sci.* 116: 33-47.

Kondo O. 2005. Regional diversity of the Ainu cranial morphology was caused by influences from the Okhotsk cultural people. In: Archaeological issue publication team on the maritime cultural exchange, editors. Sea and archaeology. Tokyo: Rokuichi-Shobo. p 233-242 (in Japanese).

Konigsberg LW. 1990. Analysis of prehistoric biological variation under a model of isolation by geographic and temporal distance. *Hum Biol.* 62:49-70.

Konigsberg LW, Kohn LAP, Cheverud JM. 1993. Cranial deformation and nonmetric trait variation. *Am J Phys Anthropol.* 90:25-48.

Lahr MM. 1996. The evolution of modern human diversity: a study of cranial variation. Cambridge: Cambridge Univ Press.

Lane RA. 1978. Non-metric osteological variation as a function of genetic kinship. *Am J Phys Anthropol.* 48:413.

Leigh SR, Konigsberg LW. 1996. Intraspecific discrete trait polymorphism in African apes: implications for variation in the fossil record. Am J Phys Anthropol Suppl 22:147.

Leigh SR, Relethford JH, Park PB, Konigsberg LW. 2004. Morphological differentiation of Gorilla subspecies. In Taylor AB, Goldsmith ML, editors. Gorilla biology: a multidisciplinary perspective. Cambridge: Cambridge University Press. p 104-131.

Liu H, Prugnolle F, Manica A, Balloux F. 2006. A geographically explicit genetic model of worldwide human-settlement history. *Am J Hum Genet.* 79:230-237.

Manica A, Prugnolle F, Balloux F. 2005. Geography is a better determinant of human genetic differentiation than ethnicity. *Hum Genet.* 118:366-371.

Manica A, Amos W, Balloux F, Hanihara T. 2007. The effect of ancient population bottlenecks on human phenotypic variation. Nature 448:346-349.

Manly BFL. 1997. Randomization, bootstrap and Monte Carlo methods in biology. Boca Raton: Chapman and Hall.

Omoto K. 1995. Genetic diversity and the origins of the 'Mongoloids'. In: Brenner S, Hanihara K, editors. The origin and past of modern human as viewed from DNA. Singapore: *World Scientific.* p 92-109.

Omoto K. Saitou N. 1997. Genetic origins of the Japanese: a partial support for the dual structure hypothesis. *Am J Phys Anthropol.* 102:437-446.

Ossenberg NS. 1981. An argument for the use of total side frequencies of bilateral non-metric skeletal traits in population distance analysis: the regression of symmetry on incidence. *Am J Phys Anthropol.* 54:471-479.

Pilbrow V. 2006. Lingual incisor traits in modern hominoids and an assessment of their utility for fossil hominoid taxonomy. *Am J Phys Anthropol.* 129:323-338

Powell JF, Neves WA. 1999. Craniofacial morphology of the first Americans: pattern and process in the peopling of the New World. *Yrbk Phys Anthropol.* 42:153-188.

Prugnolle F, Manica A, Balloux F. 2005. Geography predicts neutral genetic diversity of human populations. *Curr Biol.* 15:159-160.

Ramachandran S, Deshpande O, Roseman CC, Rosenberg NA, Feldman MW, Cavalli-Sforza LL. 2005. Support from the relationship of genetic and geographic distance in human populations for a serial founder effect originating in Africa. *Proc Natl Acad Sci USA,* 102:15942-15947.

Relethford JH. 1991. Genetic drift and anthropometric variation in Ireland. *Hum Biol.* 63:155-165.

Relethford JH. 1996. Genetic drift can obscure population history: problem and solution. *Hum Biol.* 68:29-44.

Relethford JH. 2002. Apportionment of global human genetic diversity based on craniometrics and skin color. *Am J Phys Anthropol.* 118:393-398.

Relethford JH. 2004a. Global patterns of isolation by distance based on genetic and morphological data. *Hum Biol.* 76:499-513.

Relethford JH. 2004b. Boas and beyond: migration and craniometric variation. *Am J Hum Biol.* 16:379-386.

Relethford JH. 2008. Geostatistics and spatial analysis in biological anthropology. *Am J Phys Anthropol.* 136:1-10.

Relethford JH, Blangero J. 1990. Detection of differential gene flow from patterns of quantitative variation. *Hum Bio.* 62:5-25.

Relethford,JH, Harpending HC. 1994. Craniometric variation, genetic theory, and modern human origins. *Am J Phys Anthropol.* 95:249-270.

Relethford JH, Crawford MH, Blangero J. 1997. Genetic drift and gene flow in post-famine Ireland. Hum Biol 69:443-65.

Rogers AR, Harpending HC. 1986. Migration and genetic drift in human populations. *Evolution,* 40:1312-1327.

Roseman CC, Weaver TD. 2004. Multivariate apportionment of global human craniometric diversity. *Am J Phys Anthropol.* 125:257-263.

Sardi ML, Rozzi FR, González-José R, Pucciarelli HM. 2005. South Amerindian craniofacial morphology: diversity and implications for Amerindian evolution. *Am J Phys Anthropol.* 2005:747-456.

Sato T, Amano T, Ono H, Ishida H, Kodera H, Matsumura H, Yoneda M, Masuda R. 2007. Origins and genetic features of the Okhotsk people, revealed by ancient mitochondrial DNA analysis. *J Hum Genet.* 52:18-627.

Sato T, Amano T, Ono H, Ishida H, Kodera H, Matsumura H, Yoneda M, Masuda R. 2009. Mitochondrial DNA haplogrouping of the Okhotsk people due to ancient DNA analysis: an intermediate of gene flow from the continental-Sakhalin people to the Ainu. Anthropol Sci (in press).

Scherer AK. 2007. Population structure of the classic period Maya. *Am J Phys Anthropol.* 132:367-380.

Serre D, Pääbo S. 2007. Evidence for gradients of human genetic diversity in and among continents. *Genome Res.* 14:1679-1685.

Shao J, Tu Dongsheng. 1995. The jackknife and bootstrap. New York: Springer.

Shigematsu M, Ishida H, Goto M, Hanihara T. 2004. Morphological affinities between Jomon and Ainu: reassessment based on nonmetric cranial traits. *Anthropol Sci.* 112:161-172.

Sjøvold T. A report on the heritability of some cranial measurements and non-metric traits. In: Van Vark GN, Howells WW, editors. Multivariate statistical methods in physical anthropology. Dordrecht: D Reidel Publishing Company. p 223-246.

Steadman DW. 2001. Mississippians in motion? A population genetic analysis of interregional gene flow in West-Central Illinois. *Am J Phys Anthropol.* 114:61-73.

Stojanowski CM. 2004. Population history of Native groups in pre- and postcontact Spanish Florida: aggregation, gene flow, and genetic drift on the southeastern U.S. Atlantic coast. *Am J Phys Anthropol.* 123:316-332.

Tajima A, Hayami M, Tokunaga K, Juji T, Matsuo M, Marzuki S, Omoto K, Horai S. 2004. Genetic origins of the Ainu inferred from combined DNA analyses of maternal and paternal lineages. *J Hum Genet.* 49:187-193.

Torgerson WS. 1952. Multidimensional scaling I. Theory and method. *Psychometrika,* 17:401-419.

Turner CG II. 1987. Late Pleistocene and Holocene population history of East Asia based on dental variation. *Am J Phys Anthropol.* 73:305-321.

Turner CG II. 1990. Major features of sundadonty and sinodonty, including suggestions about East Asian microevolution, population history, and late Pleistocene relationships with Australian Aboriginals. *Am J Phys Anthropol.* 82:295-317.

Von Cramon-Taubadel N, Jycett SJ. 2008. Human cranioal variation fits iterative founder effect nodel with African origin. *Am J Phys Anthropol.* 136:108-113.

Yamaguchi B. 1982. A review of the osteological characteristics of the Jomon population in prehistoric Japan. *J Anthropol Soc Nippon.* 90 (suppl):77-90.

In: Phylogeography   ISBN: 978-1-60692-954-4
Editor: Damien S. Rutgers   © 2013 Nova Science Publishers, Inc.

Chapter 5

SUTURE ZONES AND PHYLOGEOGRAPHIC CONCORDANCE: ARE THEY THE SAME AND HOW SHOULD WE TEST FOR THEIR EXISTENCE?

Nathan G. Swenson
Center for Tropical Forest Science – Asia Program
Arnold Arboretum, Harvard University
Cambridge, Massachusetts, US

ABSTRACT

Phylogeography uses present day geographic patterns of genotypes to infer the historical distribution and demography of species. While species-specific patterns have been interesting, repeated geographic patterns across species, known as phylogeographic concordance, provide evidence for general mechanisms and biogeographic events that have together shaped the distribution and diversity of genotypes. As the evidence for phylogeographic concordance started to accumulate, phylogeographers began to revisit the concept of suture zones. Suture zones, as originally described by Charles Remington, are geographic regions where multiple sister species pairs experience secondary contact and hybridize. Of interest was that some of Remington's suture zones seemed to include regions of phylogeographic concordance, suggesting that the concept and mechanisms behind the formation of suture zones could be translated from hybrid zone research to phylogeographic research. Thus, the challenge now is to explore whether a full integration of the concepts of suture zone formation and phylogeographic concordance is possible and how we should test for their existence. Here I will discuss the suture zone concept and how it relates to phylogeographic concordance, discuss previous attempts to statistically test for the existence of suture zones and phylogeographic concordance, and propose a more rigorous statistical analytical approach towards testing for the existence of suture zones and phylogeographic concordance.

THE SUTURE ZONE CONCEPT AND PHYLOGEOGRAPHIC CONCORDANCE

The present day geographic distribution of individual inter-specific hybrid zones and intra-specific phylogeographic breaks can yield insights into the past ecological, evolutionary and geographic processes that have shaped the species under study (Barton and Hewitt 1985; Avise 2000; Hewitt 2000; Hewitt 2001). By testing for the geographic concordance of several hybrid zones or phylogeographic breaks, evolutionists can discern whether the species within communities or even within entire regional biotas have been similarly influenced by historical events. Specifically, the geographic concordance between several hybrid zones or phylogeographic breaks suggests that there has been a general shared response of populations to historical events. Thus, there has been an increasing movement towards comparative analyses that ask where and why multiple hybrid zones or phylogeographic breaks occur. One striking finding emanating from many of these studies is that not only is geographic concordance frequent, but also that these spatial clusters seem to overlap substantially with suture zones (Avise 2000; Hewitt 2000; Swenson and Howard 2004; Swenson and Howard 2005).

Suture zones, as originally defined by Remington (1968), are areas where multiple hybrid zones cluster in space. In 1968 Remington produced a map containing a series of polygons that he believed represented the major and minor North American suture zones. The map was generated by compiling an extensive and, at that time, unparalleled list of known and suspected hybridizing species or subspecies pairs. The resulting suture zones were an emergent biogeographic and evolutionary pattern that demanded a general explanatory mechanism. The mechanistic hypothesis that Remington (1968) proposed was that the suture zones resulted from pervasive secondary contact of populations across all taxonomic groups that diverged while in separate glacial refugia.

Work prior to Remington (1968) had identified the tendency of hybrid zones to cluster in space (Anderson 1948, 1949; Mayr 1963). Anderson (1948, 1949) had identified several regions in the United States where plant hybrid zones tended to cluster due to intermediate environments, or niches, that were created by human disturbance, a process he termed 'hybridization of the habitat'. Hybridization of the habitat therefore was an explanatory hypothesis for the unnatural clustering of hybrid zones in space. Mayr (1963) briefly alluded to the spatial clustering of avian hybrid zones, but it is difficult to discern exactly what Mayr is referring to in several of his passages as the term 'hybrid belt' appears to be used interchangeably, as Remington (1968) notes, to refer to a single hybrid zone or a series of geographically clustered hybrid zones. While there is confusion surrounding Mayr's usage of the term hybrid belt, it seems clear that he recognized that avian hybrid zones do tend to spatially cluster and that the mechanism behind this pattern was likely secondary contact of previously isolated sister lineages. Both Mayr (1963) and Remington (1968), in agreement with Anderson (1948, 1949) did also mention the role of human modification of the environment as a pathway towards the formation of hybrid zones, but the importance of this process was downplayed in comparison to natural secondary contact. Thus, Mayr (1963) and Remington (1968) both provide the same explanatory biogeographic hypothesis for the spatial clustering of hybrid zones. Where Remington's work stands apart from Mayr's and Anderson's is the identification of hybrid zone clustering not just within birds or plants, respectively, but across many disparate taxonomic groups. Interestingly, Mayr (1970) does cite Remington (1968) on the page previous to his discussion of hybrid belts and potentially hybrid zone clustering, but the citation suggests Remington (1968) is merely a review of hybrid zones and it fails to mention the identification of hybrid zone clustering or the suture zone phenomenon.

Despite the unparalleled collection of evidence for hybrid zone clustering accumulated by Remington (1968) and the apparent importance of suture zones as general biogeographic and evolutionary phenomena, the concept of suture zones was essentially ignored for nearly three decades (Figure 1). The delayed acceptance of suture zones may have been due to several factors. First, shortly after Remington's work appeared, Lester Short responded with a scathing review (Short 1969). Short accused Remington of several wrongdoings including ignoring previous work, ignoring accepted evolutionary terminology and reporting unsubstantiated or unlikely hybrid zones particularly between avian taxa that are unlikely to be sister species (Short 1969, 1970). The use of novel terminology by Remington (1968) is perhaps excusable, but the use of non-sister species hybrid zones would weaken the case for suture zones. Uzzell and Ashmole (1970) responded to Short (1969) pointing out that non-sister species pairs do often hybridize in nature, but this argument seems to miss the point that suture zones in the strict sense should form due to the divergence of a single lineage into two lingeages while being geographically isolated and then eventually coming into secondary contact in the suture zone. Thus, some of Short's (1969) original criticisms were still salient and they may have delayed the acceptance of the suture zone concept.

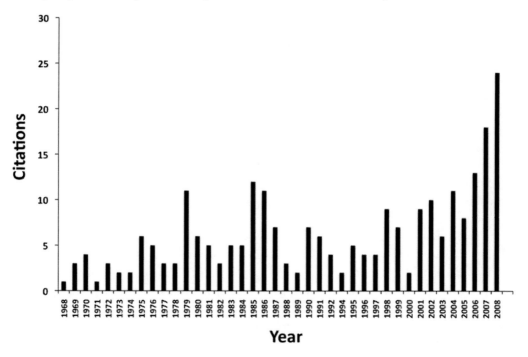

Figure 1. The number of citations of Remington (1968) over the past 40 years.

The revival of the suture zone concept in evolutionary biology can largely be attributed to Godfrey Hewitt (Hewitt 1996, 1999, 2000, 2001). The fact that Hewitt, himself a prominent hybrid zone researcher and phylogeographer, was not aware of Remington's suture zones until nearly one decade after their initial description (Hewitt 2001) only solidifies the notion that the concept of suture zones fell flat almost immediately after publication. Hewitt was able to revive interest in suture zones by repeatedly pointing towards the geographic concordance of European hybrid zones as evidence of glacial refugia and suture zones (Hewitt 1996, 1999). Hewitt's initial line of evidence for suture zones between regional biotas in Europe was later buoyed by evidence of phylogeographic concordance. Specifically, there was substantial evidence that intra-specific phylogeographic breaks also tended to spatially cluster in these exact same European suture zones (Hewitt 2000, 2001). Concurrently North American researchers were also beginning to uncover similar consistencies between Remington's suture zone map and phylogeographic concordance (Avise 2000).

It was around this time that the working definition of suture zones appeared to be informally expanded to include the spatial clustering of not just hybrid zones, but also the spatial clustering of phylogeographic breaks or phylogeographic concordance. Interestingly this more inclusive informal definition of suture zones mirrors that of the interpretation of suture zones provided by Uzzell and Ashmole (1970). Specifically, Uzzell and Ashmole (1970) argue that a suture zone should be broadly defined as the joining of two separate regional biotas where hybridization often occurs. They argued that less emphasis should be placed on whether the two populations coming into secondary contact have achieved species or sub-species status. Rather the focus should be placed on whether previously geographically isolated populations from multiple taxa are being joined or sutured in a particular geographic locality (Uzzell and Ashmole 1970). By shedding the requirement that the two populations must have diverged sufficiently while in allopatry to achieve species or sub-species status, Uzzell and Ashmole (1970) redirected the discussion regarding suture zones back towards the process of secondary contact and away from the degree of divergence achieved between the formerly sympatric populations while in allopatry. Thus, the more broadly defined suture zone concept assumed by phylogeographers is congruent with the argument of the Uzzell and Ashmole (1970). Recently, Swenson and Howard (2005) have formally modified the definition of suture zones to be the spatial clustering of hybrid zones and/or phylogeographic breaks. The argument supporting this more holistic definition of suture zone is that both hybrid zone and phylogeographic break spatial clustering are likely to result from the same biogeographic processes (Swenson and Howard 2005).

An interesting remaining conceptual issue regarding the definition of suture zones has to do with the possibility that the suturing of regional biotas may have a cyclical nature where some of the populations suturing may have only begun to diverge during the more recent glacial advance while others may have gradually diverged over several glacial advances. This type of cyclical suture zone formation seems to be particularly likely if the geographic locality of glacial refugia is consistent through time and/or abiotic gradients determine the location of suture zones (i.e. Swenson 2006). The cyclical suturing would then produce a series of secondary contacts ranging from phylogeographic breaks all the way to con-generic contact zones (Swenson and Howard 2005).

Given the above, the answer to the question of whether the spatial clustering of phylogeographic breaks, or as it is often called phylogeographic concordance, is evidence of the existence of suture zones is simple. Yes, phylogeographic concordance is indeed evidence supporting the existence of suture zones and that the definition of suture zones should formally include the clustering of phylogeographic breaks. Further, I propose that suture zones likely form cyclically with the repeated advance and retreat of glaciers. This type of cyclical suturing suggests that evidence that not all secondary contacts within a suspected suture zone that are between pairs of species, sub-species or populations that have diverged at different times (I.E. Whinnett et al. 2005) is *not* sufficient evidence to reject the existence of that suture zone nor is it sufficient evidence to reject the biogeographic processes or mechanisms that generate suture zones. Ultimately, suture zones should be expected to contain a collage of: (*i*) sister species contact zones where no hybridization occurs; (*ii*) sister species hybrid zones; and (*iii*) intra-specific phylogeographic breaks. If one or all three of these events spatially cluster in a particular geographic area, then that geographic area should be defined as a suture zone.

PREVIOUS TESTS FOR THE EXISTENCE OF SUTURE ZONES

There have been few direct tests of Remington's original suture zones. Most 'tests' of Remington's originally mapped suture zones or suspected suture zones in general have come from either qualitative assessments of overlap between phylogeographic breaks and suture zones or the documentation of phylogeographic concordance in locations not covered by Remington's original work respectively. In this section, I will first cover the two direct tests of Remington's original suture zones. I will follow this with the description of a few examples where phylogeographic concordance has been reported and the possibility that these studies have uncovered novel or supported previously reported suture zones.

While the interest in suture zones was growing during the late 1990's and early 2000's there had been no direct statistical tests for the existence of Remington's original suture zones. Swenson and Howard (2004) provided the first such test. Specifically, Swenson and Howard (2004) identified 117 hybrid zones reported in the literature from 1970 to 2002. These 117 hybrid zones occurred within the United States or Canada and had sufficient descriptions of their geographic locations that facilitated their mapping in a geographic information system (GIS). Using their GIS data base of hybrid zone locations and a digitized version of the original Remington (1968) suture zone map, Swenson and Howard (2004) asked the simple question of whether the 117 hybrid zones tended to occur in Remington's suture zones more often than expected given the percentage of the United States and Canada land area in which those suture zones occur. Surprisingly, Swenson and Howard (2004) only found minimal support for the existence of Remington's suture zones. Specifically, only the existence of two suture zones, the Great Lakes suture zone and the Rocky Mountains-Great Plains suture zone, was detected by their analyses. Thus only 2 out of the 13 major and minor suture zones were detected casting some doubt upon whether this intriguing biogeographic pattern existed at all.

The second direct test of Remington's original suture zones used a GIS to expand the Swenson and Howard (2004) hybrid zone dataset to include phylogeographic breaks and con-generic contact zones (Swenson & Howard 2005). As noted in the previous section, Remington (1968) originally defined suture zones as the clustering of hybrid zones in space. Using the argument that suture zones *sensu* Remington (1968) are perhaps too finely defined (Uzzell and Ashmole 1970) and recognizing that intra-specific phylogeographic breaks seemed to often land in Remington's suture zones by visual inspection (Avise 2000) the definition of suture zones was recast by Swenson and Howard (2005) to include the spatial clustering of hybrid zones, contact zones and phylogeographic breaks. In an effort to test whether or not phylogeographic breaks do indeed cluster in space (i.e. phylogeographic concordance), Swenson and Howard (2005) conducted a literature search for terrestrial phylogeographic breaks in North America that could be accurately mapped as points in a GIS. The point maps were then converted into two-dimensional polygons using the same methodology used by Swenson and Howard (2004) to convert hybrid point locations into a hybrid zone. This is a technique generated minimum convex polygons where the points are enclosed within a polygon that has internal angles no greater than 180 degrees. Minimum convex polygons are not affected by sampling intensity of points within a hybrid zone or phylogeographic break, are standardized and their construction is typically easy to automate inside a GIS. A spatial clustering analysis of over sixty two-dimensional phylogeographic breaks was then performed using the GIS. The specific statistic used is referred to as a Getis-Ord local G statistic (Getis and Ord 1992; Ord and Getis 1995) which identifies areas in a local-scale neighborhood that have a higher than expected value (i.e. a larger number of overlapping phylogeographic breaks) than the surrounding neighborhood. These areas are often referred to as "hotspots". This method also detects "coldspots", yet these were not analyzed. Swenson and Howard (2005) identified numerous hotspots of phylogeographic break clustering (i.e. phylogeographic concordance) in North America some of which supported previous qualitative descriptions of regions of phylogeographic concordance (e.g. Soltis et al. 1997; Walker and Avise 1998; Avise 2000). They also reported hotspots of hybrid zones, contact zones and phylogeographic breaks combined that provided greater support for the existence of Remington's suture zones than their original study that used only hybrid zones (Swenson and Howard 2004). They further supported many of the predicted glacial refugia predicted in the literature using a method originally proposed by Endler (1982). In sum this research provided perhaps the first broad-scale quantitative test of spatial clustering of phylogeographic breaks, a more rigorous test of Remington's original suture zones and identified other regions of North America that are likely to be suture zones.

There have been a number of studies that have described the concordance of many phylogeographic breaks (I.E. Soltis et al. 1997; Taberlet et al. 1998; Walker and Avise 1998; Hewitt 2000; Hewitt 2001; Soltis et al. 2006). Unfortunately, I cannot cover all of these studies in this chapter. Rather, I will cover two recent studies that have not only compiled information pertaining to the spatial clustering of phylogeographic breaks, but they have also provided the first attempts to incorporate spatial null models into this research program. The first study that will be covered in this section was recently conducted by Soltis et al. (2006). In their study, Soltis et al. compiled from the literature an extensive dataset of phylogeographic breaks in the eastern United States. The phylogeographic breaks were plotted inside a GIS and a map overlay was performed to quantify the number of phylogeographic breaks that occur in each map grid cell in their study area. The questions addressed with this analysis were: (*i*) whether the phylogeographic breaks tended to cluster in space; (*ii*) whether they were aligned similarly in space (I.E. did they all align north to south, east to west, etc.); and finally (*iii*) whether the clustering of phylogeographic breaks coincided with an abiotic gradient. Previous work by Swenson and Howard (2005) had used a Getis-Ord statistic to detect hotspots of phylogeographic break clustering. Soltis et al. (2006) improved upon this approach by introducing a spatial null modeling approach. Specifically, they wanted to determine whether the spatial patterns they observed deviated from that expected if the phylogeographic breaks were randomly distributed in their study region. To generate the null distribution against which they could compare their observed results, Soltis et al. randomly placed all of the phylogeographic breaks inside their study area maintaining only the observed shape and size of the observed phylgeographic breaks. Thus the orientation and position of the phylogeographic breaks were not maintained. This randomization was iterated multiple times and during each iteration a new random phylogeographic break clustering map was generated. Then all of the random maps were used to create the probability distribution of the number of phylogeographic breaks expected in each map grid cell. After generating their null distribution, Soltis et al. (2006) found that only one map grid cell contained a higher than expected observed number of phylgeographic breaks (I.E. phylogeographic concordance). While they found phylogeographic break clustering, the authors deemed this observed pattern to be evidence of pseudo-concordance (*sensu* Cunninghham and Collins 1994) because the orientation of the phylogeographic breaks was not uniform and they did not align with the predominant abiotic gradient in the study region, the Appalachian Mountain chain. Despite the negative result of Soltis et al. (2006), by introducing a spatial null model their study provided a quantum leap forward in the way that phylogeographers approach the question of whether phylogeographic breaks are spatially clustered. That said, the null modeling procedure used in Soltis et al. (2006) could be improved on several fronts. First, the procedure only randomized the phylogeographic breaks 20 times. The reason for this low number of iterations was due to the fact that the randomizations were performed by hand. Performing randomizations by hand is likely not a sustainable or time effective analytical approach and methods that take advantage of looping the iterations in a computer should be generated. Second, the Soltis et al. (2006) null model constained the shape and size of the observed phylogeographic breaks during the randomizations. While this is likely a robust approach, alternative null models that allow the shape of the phylogeographic break to vary should also be explored, as this approach would likely produce very different spatially random expectations. I suspect that the Soltis et al. (2006) null model is a very conservative statistical approach, but less conservative or less constrained null models may be desired and comparisons between different types of nulls should be conducted.

The second analysis of phylogeographic concordance that used a spatial null model was performed by Mortiz et al. (2009). In their study, Moritz et al. (2009) sought to determine whether a 'cryptic suture zone' exists in the Wet Tropics of northeastern Australia. The authors rightfully argued that there might be many more suture zones than those originally described by Remington (1968) and that the existence of tropical suture zones is uncertain. Moritz et al. (2009) mapped a total of 20 contact zones in their study that were determined by morphological, behavioral or genetic discordances in space. These contact zones were mapped in a GIS and latter represented as one-dimensional lines. In order to determine whether a suture zone existed in their study system the authors asked whether these 20 lines tended to cluster spatially. Specifically, they asked whether they were closer to one another than expected given a random expectation. The random expectation was derived from a spatial null model. Similar to Soltis et al. (2006), Moritz et al. (2009) represented the contact zones as lines. The difference between the two approaches was that Moritz et al. (2009) randomized the position of the contact zones only in one dimension. Due to the reduced complexity of this null modeling approach, they were able to automate this process to produce many random iterations. The reduced complexity of the null model did not hinder the study as the authors convincingly argued that their study system is essentially spatially one-dimensional. Ultimately, Moritz et al. (2009) provide the first evidence of a tropical suture zone and argue for the practical ability of suture zones to serve as natural laboratories for speciation researchers. They also successfully introduced a simple and easily automated spatial null model for testing for the existence of phylogeographic concordance and suture zones.

A NEW STASTICAL FRAMEWORK FOR DETECTING THE EXISTENCE OF SUTURE ZONES AND PHYLOGEOGRAPHIC CONCORDANCE

In a previous review (Swenson 2008), I urged phylogeographers to consider using spatial null models in their studies of phylogeographic concordance and I am excited to see this approach recently being implemented (Soltis et al. 2006; Moritz et al. 2009). These first steps towards a rigorous spatial analytical approach to testing for phylogeographic concordance and suture zones have provided a framework from which we can now expand. Specifically, a goal now is to generate spatial null models that randomize the location of phylogeographic breaks in two dimensions in an automated fashion that will allow researchers to produce thousands of random iterations. Here I argue that the tools to perform such spatial null models are already in existence, but evolutionary biologists and phylogeographers are probably unaware of them. The purpose of this section is to introduce evolutionary biologists and phylogeographers to these tools and to provide a very simplified example of how they can be used to test for the existence of phylogeographic concordance and suture zones.

For decades ecologists have tried to discern why species diversity peaks in tropical latitudes. Many of the hypotheses presented concern the latitudinal distribution of species range sizes where tropical species perhaps have smaller geographic ranges allowing for a tighter 'packing' of species and higher species diversity. The extensive ongoing debate regarding the distribution of species range sizes and species diversity provoked the development of a spatially null expectation called the Mid-Domain Effect (MDE; Colwell and Lees 2000). The MDE posits that species diversity is expected to peak in the center of a spatial domain even when species ranges are randomly distributed in space. The existence of a potential MDE in biogeography spurred the creation of novel methods to produce random species ranges in a spatially defined study region (I.E Jetz and Rahbek 2001; Rahbek et al. 2007). These methods produce random ranges by randomly throwing down a 'seed' on the study area, generally occupying one map pixel, and this seed is allowed to grow until the area covered is equivalent to the observed range size. The growth of the seed (or range) can be parametrized to be strictly spatially contiguous or it can allow for the potential to disperse and colonize non-contiguous map grid cells. The end result is a randomly generated species range that is equivalent in size to the observed range, but its shape and location does not necessarily match those of the observed range. The species ranges are then summed during each iteration to produce a map of the expected distribution of species diversity.

The original software (Jetz and Rahbek 2001) to produce these spatial null models were typically hard-coded for specific study systems and range growth syndromes (I.E. the ability to jump disperse), but newer incarnations (Rahbek et al. 2007) are much more flexible and sophisticated allowing for any size or shape of study region and the ability to constrain or loosen the restrictions on how the range can be grown in space. Here I argue that this approach can be adapted into studies of phylogeographic concordance by substituting species ranges with phylogeographic breaks and species diversity with phylogeographic break overlap. Specifically, the phylogeographer would use a map of their study region and maps of their observed phylogeographic breaks to grow random phylogeographic breaks that can be summed to produce maps of the expected phylogeographic break overlap if they were distributed randomly.

In Figures 2 and Figure 3 I present an overly simplified example of this approach that uses only three phylogeographic breaks distributed in the United States. Figure 2 shows the observed distribution of the phylogeographic breaks. Figure 3 shows the random 'seeding' and 'growth' of a phylogeographic break. The example was generated using the software BioGeoSim (http://garyentsminger.com/biogeosim/index.htm). BioGeoSim allows the researcher to quickly produce thousands of random iterations and it has a user-friendly interface making it an approach that could be quickly assimilated and utilized by the phylogeographic community. By allowing the simulation of phylogeographic breaks in two-dimensions and in an automated fashion, BioGeoSim holds the potential to quickly make investigations into phylogeographic concordance and suture zones much more rigorous and quantitative. Unfortunately, this program does not as of yet constrain the orientation of phylogeographic breaks and may have difficulty discerning phylogeographic concordance from pseudo-concordance and future generations of this software or novel software should attempt to have the option of constraining the orientation of phylogeographic breaks.

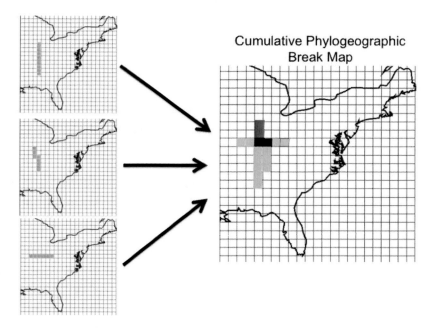

Figure 2. On the left are the three phylogeographic breaks represented as lines in this gridded map of the eastern United States. These three maps are summed together to produce the map on the right which is the sum total of the number of phylogeographic breaks that occurs in each grid cell with the darker colors representing more phylogeographic breaks being present. The objective of the spatial null modeling approach is to produce this same map, but to randomly produce the three maps on the left using the software BioGeoSim.

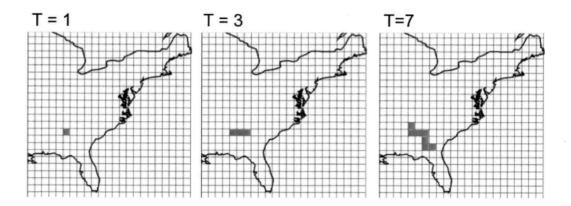

Figure 3. The simulated growth of a phylogeographic break in North America. The size of the observed phylogeographic break was seven map grid cells. The simulated break was grown for seven time steps. At each time step the break was allowed to grow in size by one grid cell in any direction. In this figure I have shown three of those time steps: Time Step 1 (T=1); Time Step 3 (T=3); and Time Step 7 (T=7). This process would be repeated for each phylogeographic break and the maps would be summed to provide the first random map of phylogeographic break clustering. This process would then be iterated hundreds to thousands of times to generate a null distribution.

CONCLUSION

This chapter sought to formally present the current definition of a suture zone and to determine whether evidence phylogeographic concordance is actually evidence for suture zones. Following in the footsteps of Uzzell and Ashmole (1970), Swenson and Howard (2005) suggested that phylogeographic concordance would be considered evidence for suture zones because both are produced from the divergence of populations while in allopatry and subsequent post-glacial recolonization and secondary contact. Here I have followed Swenson and Howard's definition, but I have formally expanded it to include the possibility that suture zones are likely cyclical due to the repeated advance and retreat of glaciers. Specifically, suture zones likely contain recently and anciently divergent sister lineages coming into contact and evidence of either lends support to the importance of glacial refugia in producing species and phylogenetic diversity.

Tests for the existence of suture zones have been rare, while tests for phylogeographic concordance have been more common. In the past (Swenson 2008) and presently I have argued that the spatial analyses in these studies could be vastly improved by incorporating spatial null models. I have highlighted two recent studies that have successfully taken on this challenge, but there is room for improvement. In response, I have outlined how a null modeling approach used in ecology that simulates species ranges can be utilized in the field of phylogeography. It is my hope that phylogeographers will begin to utilize this particular approach and more refined spatial null modeling approaches in the future to support their inferences regarding suture zones and phylogeographic concordance. The field of phylogeography has benefited from the outstanding advances in genetics and through the use of more explicit quantitative spatial analyses it will also benefit from the contributions of fields like spatial ecology and geography.

ACKNOWLEDGMENTS

I thank Dan Howard for introducing me to the concept of suture zones. I thank Walter Jetz and Nick Gotelli for their help and advice in regards to the spatial null modeling discussed in this chapter. I was supported by a National Science Foundation Postdoctoral Fellowship in Bioinfomatics.

REFERENCES

Anderson, E. 1948. Hybridization of the habitat. *Evolution* 2:1-9.

Anderson, E. 1949. *Introgressive Hybridization*. Wiley, New York.

Avise, J.C. 2000. *Phylogeography: The History and Formation of Species*. Harvard University Press, Cambridge, Massachusetts.

Barton, N.H., and G.M. Hewitt. 1985. Analysis of hybrid zones. *Annual Review of Ecology and Systematics* 16:113-148.

Colwell, R.K., and D.C. Lees. 2000. The mid-domain effect: geometric constraints on the geography of species richness. *Trends in Ecology and Evolution* 15:70-76

Cunningham, C.W., and T.M. Collins. 1994. Developing model systems for molecular biogeography: vicariance and interchange in marine invertebrates. In *Molecular Ecology and Evolution: Approaches and Applications* (Eds. Schierwater, B., B. Streit, P. Wagner, and R. DeSalle) pp. 405-433. Birkhauser Verlag, Basel, Switzerland.

Endler, J.A. 1982. Pleistocene forest refuges: fact or fancy? In: *Biological Diversification in the Tropics* (Ed. Prance, G.T.) pp. 641-657. Columbia University Press, New York.

Getis, A., and J.K. Ord. 1992. The analysis of spatial association by use of distance statistics. *Geographic Analysis* 24:189-206.

Hewitt, G.M. 1996. Some genetic consequences of ice ages, and their role in divergence and speciation. *Biological Journal of the Linnean Society* 58:247-276.

Hewitt, G.M. 1999. Post-glacial recolonization of European Biota. *Biological Journal of the Linnean Society* 68:87-112.

Hewitt, G.M. 2000. The genetic legacy of the Quaternary ice ages. *Nature* 405:907-913.

Hewitt, G.M. 2001. Speciation, hybrid zones and phylogeography – or seeing genes in space and time. *Molecular Ecology* 10:537-549.

Jetz, W., and C. Rahbek. 2001. A two-dimensional geometric constraints model explains much of the species richness pattern in African birds. *Proceedings National Academy of Science of the U.S.A.* 98:5661-5666.

Mayr, E. 1963. *Animal Species and Evolution*. Harvard University Press, Cambridge, Massachusetts.

Mayr, E. 1970. *Populations, Species, and Evolution*. Harvard University Press, Cambridge, Massachussetts.

Moritz, C., C.J. Hoskin, J.B. MacKenzie, B.L. Phillips, M. Tonione, N. Silva, J. VanDerWal, S.E. Williams and C.H. Graham. 2009. Identification and dynamics of a cryptic suture zone in tropical rainforest. *Proceedings of the Royal Society of London Series B.* 276:1235-1244.

Ord, J.K., and A. Getis. 1995. Local spatial autocorrelation statistics: distributional issues and an application. *Geographic Analysis* 27:286-306.

Rahbek, C., N.J. Gotelli, R.K. Colwell, G.L. Entsminger, T.F.L.V.B. Rangel, and G.R. Graves. 2007. Predicting continental-scale patterns of bird species richness with spatially explicit models. *Proceedings of the Royal Society of London Series B.* 274:165-174.

Remington, C.L. 1968. Suture-zones of hybrid interaction between recently joined biotas. In: *Evolutionary Biology* (Eds. Dobzhansky T, Hecht MK, Steere WC) pp. 321-428. Appleton-Century-Crofts, New York.

Short, L.L. 1969. "Suture-zones," secondary contacts, and hybridization. *Systematic Zoology* 18:458-460.

Short, L.L. 1970. A reply to Uzzell and Ashmole. *Systematic Zoology* 19:199-202.

Soltis, D.E., M.A. Gitzendanner, D.D. Strenge, and P.A. Soltis. 1997. Chloroplast DNA intraspecific phylogeography of plants from the Pacific Northwest of North America. Plant Systematics and Evolution 206:353-373.

Soltis, D.E., A.B. Morris, J.S. McLachlan, P.S. Manos, and P.S. Soltis. 2006. Comparative phylogeography of unglaciated eastern North America. *Molecular Ecology* 15:4261-4293

Swenson, N.G. 2006. GIS-based niche models reveal unifying climatic mechanisms that maintain the location of avian hybrid zones in a North American suture zone. *Journal of Evolutionary Biology* 19:717-725.

Swenson, N.G. 2008. The past and future influence of geographic information systems on hybrid zone, phylogeographic and speciation research. *Journal Evolutionary Biology* 21:421-434.

Swenson, N.G., and D.J. Howard. 2004. Do suture zones exist? *Evolution* 58:2391-2397.

Swenson, N.G., and D.J. Howard. 2005. Clustering of contact zones, hybrid zones, and phylogeographic breaks in North America. *American Naturalist* 166:581-591.

Taberlet, P., L. Fumagalli, A. Wust-Saucy, and J. Cosson. 1998. Comparative phylogeography and postglacial colonization routes in Europe. *Molecular Ecology* 8:1923-1934.

Uzzell, T., and N.P. Ashmole. 1970. Suture-zones: an alternative view. *Systematic Zoology* 19:197-199.

Walker, D., and J.C. Avise. 1998. Principles of phylogeography as illustrated by freshwater and terrestrial turtles in the southeastern United States. *Annual Review of Ecology and Systematics* 29:23-58.

Whinnett, A., M. Zimmerman, K.R. Willmott, N. Herrera, R. Mallarino, F. Simpson, M. Joron, G. Lamas, and J. Mallet. 2005. Strikingly variable divergence times inferred across an Amazonian butterfly 'suture zone'. *Proceedings of the Royal Society of London Series B.* 272:2525-2533.

In: Phylogeography
Editor: Damien S. Rutgers

ISBN: 978-1-60692-954-4
© 2013 Nova Science Publishers, Inc.

Chapter 6

DIFFERENTIATION HISTORY OF DRAGONFLIES IN THE INSULAR EAST ASIA REVEALED BY THE GENE GENEALOGY (ODONATA: HEXAPODA)

Takuya Kiyoshi[*]

Center for Ecological Research, Kyoto University
Hirano, Otsu, Shiga, Japan

ABSTRACT

The insular East Asia contains many islands encompasses various climatic regions, from subtropical to subarctic. Its fauna contains about 400 species of the order Odonata (dragonflies and damselflies), including many endemic ones. Two groups of dragonflies, the genus *Davidius* and *Anotogaster sieboldii* show interesting radiation patterns in this region. Both the mitochondrial and nuclear gene genealogy revealed that four species of the genus *Davidius* in this region seem to have diversified through the geographical connection and disconnection between the Korean Peninsula and Japanese main islands. The habitat of the larvae of *D. moiwanus* sspp. were estimated to have shifted from rivers to narrow streams in wetlands. Molecular phylogeographical analyses revealed not only their divergence history in the insular region but also including the process divided them from the continental congeners. Mitochondrial gene genealogy based on COI gene sequence data revealed that *A. sieboldii* includes two deeply differentiated clades that seem to have diverged in late Miocene or early Plicocene. Each of these two clades includes three inner clades that seem to have differentiated in Pleistocene.

---

[*] Telephone: (+77)-549-8215
Fax: (+77)-549-8201
E-mail: kiyoshi@ecology.kyoto-u.ac.jp

INTRODUCTION

The insular East Asia contains many islands that range from the subarctic to the subtropical. Since the geographical formation of this region in the middle Miocene (Ichikawa *et al.*, 1970; Yonekura *et al.*, 2001), extensive geographical and climatic changes have contributed to the biotic exchange and diversification of this region. The fauna of the insular East Asia contains about 400 species of the order Odonata (dragonflies and damselflies), including many endemic taxon (Tsuda, 2000). Moreover, geographical variations are often observed among the insular populations. The history of their divergence often seems to have been closely related to the geographical formation process of these islands. For the Japanese main islands, there are fairly good geographical information on its formation history (*e.g.*, Ichikawa *et al.*, 1970; Yonekura *et al.*, 2001) but the detail of the insularization process of the Ryukyu Archipelago has not been so clear. It sometimes causes difficulty in calibrating divergence timing of phylogenetic divergence because the margins of the errors of the estimated timings of geographical changes are so wide. It should be carefully considered of the propriety of geographical information like the timing of insularization in Ryukyu Archipelago.

With advances and spread of molecular biological techniques, phylogeographical analyses on the many kind of creatures distributed in this area revealed the history of their speciation or population differentiation. In this region, reviews on phylogeographic studies on some groups have published in this decade, for example, reptiles and amphibians (Ota, 1998), fish (Watanabe *et al.*, 2006), and carabid beetles (Osawa *et al.*, 2002)).

Two groups of dragonfly (*Davidius* and *Anotogaster sieboldii*) in this region show interesting patterns and processes of differentiation. Molecular phylogeographical analyses revealed not only their divergence history in the insular region but also including the processes that divided them from the continental congeners. What is more, the habitat shift process of the larvae in the genus *Davidius*, from streams to wetlands, was clearly inferred from both the mitochondrial and nuclear gene genealogy. In this chapter, I will not only try to make review of these individual studies but also to introduce some of interesting patterns in this region that have not still phylogeographically understood.

CASE I—DIFFERENTIATION PROCESS OF THE GENUS *DAVIDIUS* IN THE INSULAR EAST ASIA

The genus *Davidius* includes about 20 species distributed in the East to South-East Asia (Tsuda, 2000). In the insular region of East Asia, three species are distributed in Japanese main islands and adjacent ones: *D. nanus, D. moiwanus* and *D. fujiama* (Asahina and Inoue, 1973; Ishida *et al.*, 1988; see also, Figure 1). One other *Davidius* species, *D. lunatus*, is distributed in the Korean Peninsula, Northern region of China and a part of Siberia (Asahina, 1989; Bartenef, 1914; Zhao, 1990; See also, Figure 1). The distribution area of these four species seems to be isolated from other members of this genus (Zhao, 1990), and no *Davidius* species are distributed in Taiwan, Ryukyu Archipelago and in most part of Siberia. The ancestral population of Japanese *Davidius* species likely colonized Japan from the Korean Peninsula.

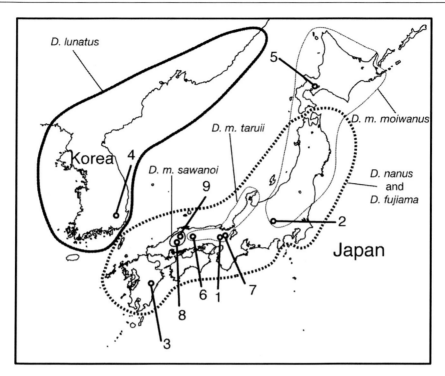

After Kiyoshi and Sota (2006).

Figure 1. Geographic distribution and sample localities of the four *Davidius* species. See Table 1 for locality names corresponding to the numbers on the map.

In the three species distributed in Japan, larval habitat usages are different in each species. The larvae of *D. moiwanus* inhabit narrow wetland streams in Honshu, and both wetland streams and rivers in Hokkaido, where no other *Davidius* species occurs (Ishida *et al.*, 1988; Sugimura *et al.*, 1999).

To infer the divergence history of the genus *Davidius* in the insular East Asia, the molecular phylogenetic trees were reconstructed based on the mitochondrial and nuclear sequence data (Kiyoshi and Sota, 2006). In the phylogeographic analyses using mitochondrial genes, sequences encompassing 721 bp of COI, 62 to 64 bp of leucine transfer RNA (tRNA), and 36 bp of COII were directly sequenced. The maximum likelihood and Bayesian analyses on mitochondrial sequence data resulted in a topology that did not support the monophyly of *D. moiwanus* (Figure 2a). These analyses suggested that *D. nanus* and *D. moiwanus* are sister to *D. lunatus* and that these three species form a monophyletic group with respect to *D. fujiama*. Of the three *D. miwanus* subspecies, *D. m. moiwanus* showed difference from *D. m. taruii* and *D. m. sawanoi*. On the other hand, the latter two subspecies did not exhibit reciprocal monophyly.

To infer the nuclear gene genealogy, about 1100 bp of ITS sequence that encompasses ITS1, 5.8S ribosomal RNA (rRNA), and ITS2 was directly sequenced. Ten alleles were obtained from *Davidius* samples. In the reconstructions of the mitochondrial gene genealogy, *Lanthus fujiacus* were used as outgroup but its ITS sequence could not be obtained for an unknown reason. Although the ITS regions showed high variability, sequence variation within populations as well as among populations within subspecies or species was rather low.

Tree searches by the direct optimization (Wheeler, 1996) revealed *D. moiwanus* monophyly, with *D. nanus* sister to *D. moiwanus* (Figure 2b). Within *D. moiwanus*, *D. m. moiwanus* was monophyletic and the western subspecies *D. m. sawanoi* and *D. m. taruii* formed another clade. Each of the latter two subspecies was also monophyletic; two *D. m. taruii* populations exhibited only one allele. The direct optimization for the combined data of COI and ITS also showed the monophyly of *D. miwanus*.

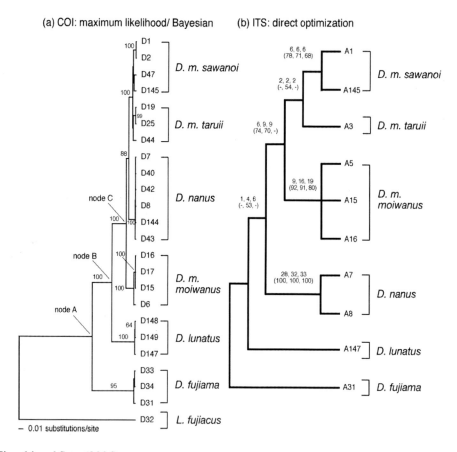

After Kiyoshi and Sota (2006).

Figure 2. (a) Maximum-likelihood tree with molecular clock assumption. The numerals above the branches are the posterior probabilities (percentages) of nodes shoared with the 50% majority-rule consensus tree resulting from Bayesian analysis. Nodes A, B, and C were considered in the estimation of divergence times. (b) Strict consensus of direct optimization analyses of the ITS data set. The results were identical for three gap/change cost settings. Numerals above the branches: Bremer support values, with jackknife percentages (when >50%) in parentheses, from direct optimization. Triplet numerals are for gap/change costs of 1:1, 2:1, and 3:1, respectively.

Although analysis of mitochondrial DNA sequence data did not clearly reveal the monophyly of *D. moiwanus*, nuclear DNA sequence data did. Species-level polyphyly or paraphyly is a common phenomenon for gene genealogies, especially those of mitochondrial genes (*e.g.*, Funk and Omland, 2003; Ballard and Whitelock, 2004). Theoretically, This paraphyly can result from incomplete or random lineage sorting and introgressive hybridization. This results suggest that three groups (*D. nanus, D. moiwanus moiwanus* and

D. m. taruii + D. m. sawanoi) differentiated over a short time, which could lead to an ambiguous differentiation pattern because the sequence divergence between *D. nanus* and *D. moiwanus* subspecies is large and there has been no evidence of interspecific hybridization, the effects of introgressive hybridization could be excluded.

Ecological Differentiation

The larvae of *D. nanus, D. fujiama,* and *D. lunatus* inhabit rivers. However, larvae of *D. moiwanus* inhabit narrow wetland streams in Honshu, and both wetland streams and rivers in Hokkaido, where no other *Davidius* species occurs (Ishida *et al.,* 1988; Sugimura *et al.,* 1999)

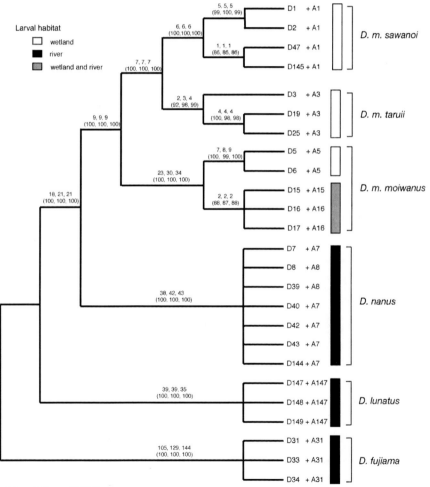

After Kiyoshi and Sota (2006).

Figure 3. Strict consensus of direct optimization analyses of the combined COI+ITS data set. Results were identical for the three gap/change cost settings. The combination of COI haplotype and ITS allele is indicated at the terminal node (See Table 1 for haplotype/allele codes). Numerals above branches: Bremer support values, with jackknife percentages in parentheses, from direct optimization analyses. Triplet numerals are for gap/change costs of 1:1, 2:1, and 3:1, respectively. Larval habitats are indicated by baras beside the taxon names.

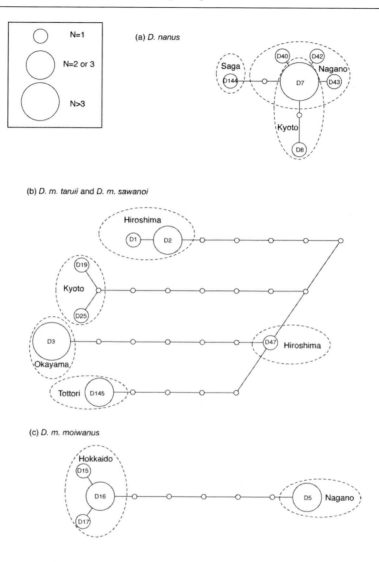

After Kiyoshi and Sota (2006).

Figure 4. Statistical parsimony tree of the haplotypes from *D. nanus* and *D. moiwanus*. Haplotypes are indicated by large open circles with haplotype codes (See Table 1 and Figureure 2). Mutational steps are represented by thick lines with small open circles representing intermediate haplotypes that did not appear in the samples. Haplotypes from the same locality are encircled by a dashed line, with the locality number indicated (See Table 1).

The phylogenetic hypothesis resulting from the combined data of COI and ITS (Figure 3) suggests that the riverine habitat is ancestral larval habitat of *Davidius* and the wetland habitat is derived. Part of the ancestral population (ancestral *D. moiwanus*) may have adapted to wetlands, and subsequently, the range of the riverine type (ancestral *D. nanus*) may have extended to encompass localized wetlands. The recent range expansion by *D. nanus* is supported by the low sequence divergence over the distribution range compared to that of *D. moiwanus* (Figure 4).

Davidius nanus and *D. fujiama* deposit eggs in the surface waters of rivers, co-occurring over a wide range in Japan. Although further field study is needed for their habitat use, adult *D. nanus* emerge in the middle reach of the river, far below their oviposition sites, whereas *D. fuujiama* emerge not far below the oviposition sites. Moreover, *D. nanus* reproduce earlier than *D. fujiama* (Ishida *et al.*, 1988; Odonatological Society of Osaka, 1998). *Davidius lunatus* occurs only in Korea and Primorsky Krai, Russia. Therefore, a detailed study of its larval habitat use is indispensable to understand the extent of the *Davidius* riverine niche in the absence of other sympatric species.

Timing of Divergence Inferred From COI Sequence Data

The maximum likelihood tree with the molecular-clock assumption did not differ statistically from the tree without assumption. The former was used to estimate divergence times (Figure 2a). To calibrate age, the branching between *D. fujiama* and the other three species (Figure 2a; node A) was assumed to be 2.5 Ma. With this calibration, the branching between *D. lunatus* and *D. nanus* + *D. moiwanus* (node B) represents 1.92±0.01 (mean ± SE) Ma, and differentiation within the *D. nanus* + *D. moiwanus* lineage (node C) occurred after 0.77±0.04 Ma. Alternatively, if node B were assumed to be 3.5Ma, node A would represent 6.37±0.03 Ma, and node C would represent 1.41±0.07 Ma.

The gene genealogies suggest that the continental *Davidius* lineage colonized Japan at least twice; the first colonizer was the ancestor of *D. fujiama*; the second was the ancestor of *D. nanus* and *D. moiwanus*. If, however, the four *Davidius* species studied here are monophyletic, it is also possible that the ancestor of the four species colonized Japan, and the ancestor of *D. lunatus* migrated from Japan to the continent. These two hypotheses require two dispersal/colonization events and are equally parsimonious reconstruction of the historical biogeography. We cannot determine which is the most likely hypothesis because we could not examine continental *Davidius* species other than *D. lunatus*. In either case, we can assume that the Tsushima Strait has acted as the major geographic barrier promoting differentiation of the continental and Japanese lineages.

Since no fossil record is available to calibrate the COI sequence divergence of *Davidius*, we assumed that either of two nodes that led to *D. fujiama* and *D. lunatus* corresponds to the time when the western channel (Tsushima Strait) of the Sea of Japan opened 3.5 Ma (Tada, 1994). The Tsushima Strait was closed from 10 to 3.5 Ma (Tada, 1994); during this period, faunal exchange between the continent and Japan would have been frequent. After 3.5 Ma, the Tsushima Strait was open except from 2.5 to 1.7 Ma and later regression periods during glacial ages (Iijima and Tada, 1990; Tada, 1994; Kitamura *et al.*, 2001).

The estimated substitution rate for mitochondrial DNA sequence data of insects, including the COI region, ranges from 1.5% (Farrell, 2001; Quek *et al.*, 2004) to 2.3% (Brower, 1994) per million years. The uncorrected pair-wise sequence difference at node A (Figure 2a) is 11.0±0.3% (mean±SD), implying a substitution rate of 3.1% per million years, which is much faster than previously reported. When node B (Figure 2a) is assumed to be 3.5 Ma, the substitution rate is 2.3% (uncorrected pair-wise sequence divergence, 7.7±0.2%), equal to the highest proposed rate. Under this assumption, the *D. fujiama* lineage that gave rise to *D. lunatus*, *D. nanus* and *D. moiwanus* may have existed in Japan in the Pliocene. At present, we have no evidence to support either calibration. However, either calibration yields estimated divegence times for the *D.nanus* + *D. moiwanus* clade in the Pleistocene (1.4-0.8Ma). Differentiation among *D. nanus* and *D. moiwanus* subspecies was likely promoted by the rapid changes in climate and geography in Japan during the Pleistocene.

CASE II—DIVERGENCE HISTORY OF *ANOTOGASTER SIEBOLDII* (SELYS, 1854)

A golden-ringed dragonfly, *Anotogaster sieboldii* (Selys, 1854), is distributed widely in the insular East Asia and partly in the continental area (Tsuda, 2000). This species contains some geographical variations, at least three population groups could be distinguished morphologically (Ishida et al., 1988; Asahina, 1989; Wang, 2000): the first from Japanese main and adjacent islands and Korean Peninsula, the second from Central Ryukyus (Okinawajima and Amamioshima) and the third from the Yaeyama Group (Iriomotejima and Ishigakijima) and Taiwan. The information on its distributed area in China is still insufficient. The phylogenetic analyses among 18 populations (Figure 5), including some Chinese populations, were conducted, and thereby inferred the coloniazation and differentiation of the species by Kiyoshi (2008).

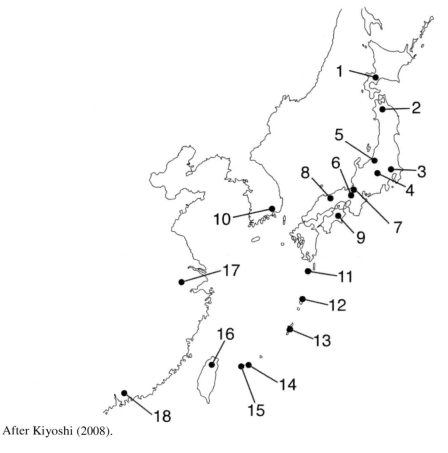

After Kiyoshi (2008).

Figure 5. Sampling localities of *Anotogaster sieboldii*. See Table 1 for the locality numbers in the map.

Mitochondrial gene genealogy was estimated by the maximum likelihood method and Bayesian inference (Figure 6) based on the partial sequence data of COI and COII genes (541 and 304 bp, respectively). It revealed that *Anotogaster sievoldii* involves two deeply separated clades that were confirmed to be monophyletic. One of them includes three inner clades; the first from Japanese main islands, Korean Peninsula and Yakushima (northern area, hereafrter), the second from Amamioshima and the third from Okinawajima. The second and the third ones were reveled to be a sister group. The other major clade involves the populations of the Yaeyama Group (Iriomotejima and Ishigajima), Taiwan and East China. The populations of the Yaeyama Grouup and Taiwan were reconstructed as reciprocal monophyletic groups.

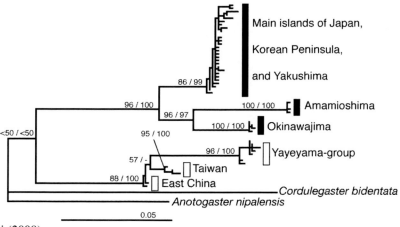

After Kiyoshi (2008).

Figure 6. Maximum-likelihood tree. Former numerals above the branches are bootstrap percentages (when >50%) in parentheses. The latter numerals separated by / above the branches are the posterior probabilities (percentages) of nodes in Bayesian analysis except for the node that did not apearr in the Bayesian analysis (shown as -).

Subdivided Ppulations

The relationship among the populations of *A. sieboldii* haplotypes was represented using statistical parsimony networks (Figure 7). The five networks were disconnected beyond the 95% confidence limit: (1) northern populations, (2) Amamioshima, (3) Okinawajima, (4) Taiwan and the East China and (5) Yaeyama Group, respectively.

The population differentiation test (Raymond and Rousset, 1995) between the populations of Kyoto, Hokkaido and Korea detected significant difference for each pair (p < 0.05). Although the Yakushima population possessed two original haplotypes (AS104 and AS108; see Figure 7 (a) and Table 1), the insufficiency of sampling (n=2) caused difficulty in applying population differentiation tests. The population of Amamioshima and Okinawajima (Figure 7(b), (c), respectively) showed relatively low genetic diversity as compared to northern populations (Figure 7(a)). Haplotypes of Taiwanese and East Chinese samples were connected (Figure 7(d)) but further sampling would be needed to examine population differentiation. Two populations of the Yaeyama Group shared some haplotypes between each other (Table 1; see also Figure 7(e)) but the exact test was significant (p < 0.05).

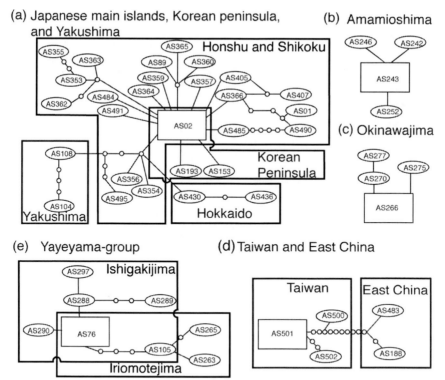

After Kiyoshi (2008).

Figure 7. Statistical parsimony networks of the haplotypes of *Anotogaster sieboldii*. Haplotypes are indicated by large open circles with haplotype codes (see Table 2). Mutational steps are represented by thick lines with small open circles representing intermediate haplotypes that did not appear in the samples.

Table 1. Specimens used in the phylogenetic analysis and haplotype/allele codes of COI and ITS sequences

Locality[a]	Taxon	COI haplotype (n)[b]	ITS allele (n)[b]
1. Kyoto	*Davidius nanus* (Selys)	D7(1), D8(1)	A7 (1), A8 (1)
	D. fujiama Fraser	D31(1), D33(1), D34(1)	A31 (3)
	Lanthus fujiacus (Fraser)	D32(1)	---
2. Nagano	*D. nanus* (Selys)	D7(2), D40(1), D42(1),D43(1)	A7 (4), A8 (1)
	D. moiwanus moiwanus (Okumura)	D5(1), D6(1)	A5 (2)
3. Saga	*D. nanus* (Selys)	D144(1)	A7 (1)
4. Busan	*D. lunatus* (Bartenef)	D147(1), D148(1), D149(1)	A147 (3)
5. Hokkaido	*D. m. moiwanus* (Okumura)	D15(1), D16(2), D17(1)	A15 (1), A16 (3)
6. Okayama	*D. m. taruii* Asahina et Inoue	D44(4)	A3 (4)
7. Kyoto	*D. m. taruii* Asahina et Inoue	D19(1), D25(1)	A3 (2)
8. Hiroshima	*D. m. sawanoi* Asahina et Inoue	D1(1), D2(2), D47(1)	A1 (4)
9. Tottori	*D. m. sawanoi* Asahina et Inoue	D145(2)	A145 (2)

[a] Locality numbers are those used in Figure 1.

[b] Haplotype/allele codes correspond to those used in Figures 2-4

Differentiation Hstory of A. sieboldii

The timing of genetic divergence was inferred by using the estimated substitution rate for insect mitochondrial DNA sequence data because there have been no fossil records on this species, and geographical information on the formation of the insular East Asia have been insufficient to calibrate the timing. The rate ranges from 1.5% [uncorrected pair-wise distance (p-distance); Farrell 2001; Quek *et al.,* 2004] to 2.3% (Brower, 1994) per million years.

Table 2. Specimens used in the phylogenetic analyses and haplotype codes of COI sequences

Species	Locality[a]	No. specimens	Haplotype No (n)[b]
Anotogaster sieboldii	1. Sapporo, Hokakido, Japan	12	AS427 (11), AS436 (1)
	2. Aomori, Honshu, Japan	1	AS02 (1)
	3. Saitama, Honshu, Japan	7	AS02 (1), AS484 (1), AS485 (1), AS490 (1), AS491 (2), AS495 (1)
	4. Nagano, Honshu, Japan	2	AS02 (1), AS405 (1)
	5. Nigata, Honshu, Japan	1	AS02 (1)
	6. Kyoto, Honshu, Japan	18	AS01 (1), AS02 (5), AS353 (1) AS354 (1), AS355 (1), AS356 (1), AS357 (1), AS359 (1), AS360 (1), AS362 (1), AS363 (1), AS364 (1), AS365 (1), AS366 (2)
	7. Fukui, Honshu, Japan	1	AS407 (1)
	8. Tottori, Honshu, Japan	1	AS89 (1)
	9. Ehime, Shikoku, Japan	2	AS02 (2)
	10. Busan, Korea	13	AS02 (11), AS153 (1), AS193 (1)
	11. Yakushima, Japan	2	AS104 (1), AS108 (1)
	12. Amamioshima, Japan	12	AS242 (2), AS243 (8), AS246 (1), AS252 (1)
	13. Okinawajima Japan	15	AS266 (11), AS270 (1), AS275 (1), AS277 (1)
	14. Ishigakijima, Japan	20	AS76 (3), AS105 (1), AS287 (1), AS288 (12), AS289 (1),AS290 (1),AS297 (1)
	15. Iriomotejima, Japan 5		AS76 (2), AS105 (1), AS263 (1), AS265 (1)
	16. Taipei, Taiwan	3	AS500 (1), AS501 (1), AS502 (1)
	17. Hangzhou, China	1	AS188 (1)
	18. Guandong, China	1	AS483 (1)
Anotogaster nipalensis	Nepal	1	AS151 (1)
Cordulegaster bidentata	Romania	2	AS131 (2)

[a]Locality numbers are those used in Figure 5.
[b]Haplotype codes correspond to those used in Figure 6–7.

The genetic divergence of the two highly divergent mitochondrial lineages in *A. sieboldii* (10.0% ± 0.9%, p-distance ± SE) corresponds to the timing of 7.3 to 4.0 Ma. They seem to have differentiated in late Miocene or early Plicocene. It would be probably before the formation of the insular East Asia (Machida *et al.*, 2001).

The sequence divergence between the two population groups of the Central Ryukyus (Okinawajima and Amamioshima) and the northern region (5.6% ± 0.7%) corresponds to the timing of 2.1 to 4.2 Myr. For the major clade including samples from northern area, Amamioshima and Okinawajima, their divergence occurred in the Pleistocene. Firstly, the opening of the Tokara-Gap in early Pleistocene (Kizaki and Oshiro, 1980; Ota, 1998) might have been separated these population groups. Subsequently populations of Okinawajima and Amamioshima would have been divided.

In the northern populations, only endemic haplotypes were found in populations of Hokkaido and Yakushima, and a common haplotype (AS02) was distributed in the Korean Peninsula and other Japanese main islands (Figure 7(a) and Table 1). The populations of Hokkaido and Yakushima might have been isolated before the population subdivision between other Japanese main islands and Korean Peninsula.

The other major clade includes populations of the Yaeyama Group (Iriomotejima and Ishigakijima), Taiwan and East China. The sequence divergence between populations of East China and Taiwan (1.3 ± 0.3%) ranges from 0.4 to 1.1 Myr. The genetic distance between populations of Yaeyama Group and Taiwan (4.7 ± 0.7%) corresponds to 1.7 to 3.6 Ma. These populations might have been segregated by the opening of the straits in Pleistocene (Kizaki and Oshiro, 1980; Ota, 1998). The subdivision between populations of Ishigakijima and Iriomotejima would have occurred later.

INTERESTING PATTERNS OF DISTRIBUTION IN THEINSULAR EAST ASIA

Most of the Odonata fauna in the insular East Asia have not been phylogeographically researched. In this section, I want to mention on two especially interesting patterns of distribution that also still need phylogeographic investigations.

Case I—Isolated Distribution wth Facing Each Other Across Closely Related Species

In the Ryukyu archipelago, at least, two taxon show similar interesting patterns of distribution. The genus *Hemicordulia* includes two species distributed in this insular region. *H. okinawensis* Asahina, 1947 distributed in Central Ryukyus (Okinawajima and Amamioshima). The distribution area of its congener *H. mindana nipponica* Asahina, 1980 is facing each other across that of *H. okinawensis* (See also, Figure 8(a)).

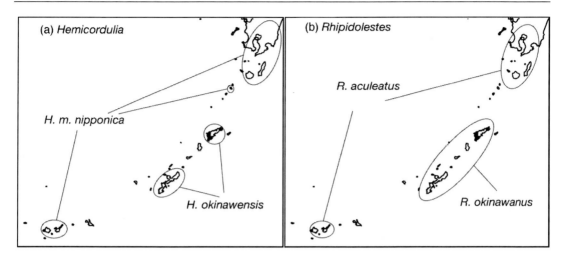

Figure 8. Geographic distribution patterns. (a) *Hemicordulia*. (b) *Rhipidolestes*.

In this case, both of the species, *H. m. nipponica* and *H. okinawensis*, have not been recorded from continent. Without assumption of over sea dispersals of the ancestral populations of *H. m. nipponica* into northern area (Nakanoshima, Tanegashima and southern part of Kyushu) or of the extinction of *H. m. nipponica* in Central Ryukyus, it could not be explained this distribution pattern.

One another similar pattern has found in the genus *Rhipidolestes*. *R. aculeatus sakishimanus* Asahina, 1993 distributed in Yaeyama group, *R. a. yakusimensis* Asahina, 1951 distrubuted in Yakushima and southern part of Kyushu. Between these regions, from Amamioshima to Okinawajima, *R. okinawanus* Asahina, 1951 were recorded (See also, Figure 8(b)). The distributed areas of *R. acuuleatus* are clearly isolated with being immediately distributed area of *R. okinawanus*. This distribution pattern also needs almost the same kind of assumptions as the case of the genus *Hemicordulia* because none of these two species are recorded from the continent.

These two genera seem to share the strange pattern of distribution. It would be preferable to compare the phylogenetic relation ships among populations in each species. From the viewpoint of comparative phylogeography, if the gene genealogies of each species show very similar topology, it would suggest us a existence of the past geographic changes that caused these distribution pattern.

Case II—Living Fossil Dragonfly

Usually extant Odonata are divided into 3 suborders, Anisoptera (dragonflies), Zygoptera (damselfly) and Anisozygoptera. In the last suborder, there has been only two extant species known. *Epiophlebia laidlawi* Tillyard, 1921 are from Himalaya, and *E. superstes* (Selys, 1889) are from Japanese mainislands. There are some fossils belong to this subfamily but now only these two species are known extant members.

The genus *Epiophlebia* is very important not only from the viewpoint of the phylogeography of Odonata but also for the understanding of the evolution of Odonata. This taxon possess wings resembles (or shares) the characters of damselflies, and there body are like dragonflies. Therefore, they have been thought to be a key taxon to understand the diversification of Odonata.

CONCLUSION

In this chapter, I tried to make review two phylogeographic researches of dragonflies in the insular East Asia. Dragonflies in this region have many unopened phylogeographical problems. Especially, Ryukyu archipelago involves many endemic taxon, or populations that are differentiated from other region. Dragonflies are usually thought to possess great ability of flying. Some species easily make over-sea dispersals (*e.g. Pantala flavescene* (Fabricius, 1798), *Sympetrum depressiusculum* (Selys, 1841) and *S. cordulegaster* (Selys, 1883)) but populations of many species distributed in this insular region seem to have differentiated in rather old age. In this region, there are still many groups of Odonata left to be phylogeographically understood. To infer the diversification history of dragonflies in this region, it would be needed to compare the differentiation process of each group.

Some of the endangered species or populations, possibly threatened by the activity of human beings, throw us problems of great urgency. In planning the conservation of insular populations in endangered state, if abundant populations of the same species are distributed in other region (continent or other neighbor islands) without necessity for their protection, it could be controversial. Some researchers may insist on the conservation of distinct populations because of their endemism but others may reject the need of their preservation because "species" itself is not in endangered state. In the case of the species distributed in the insular East Asia, this kind of problem sometimes occurred. In my opinion, it might be preferable to adopt the concept of the evolutionary significant unit (Ryder, 1986), especially on the insular populations. In the future, advances in phylogeography of Odonata in the insular East Asia would reveal the genetic population differentiation of many species.

REFERENCES

Asahina, S. (1989) The Odonata of Korean Peninsula, a summarized review. Part II. Anisoptera 1 (Gomphidae). Gekkan-Mushi, 222, 8–13.

Asahina, S. & Inoue, K. (1973) Descriptions of two new geographical races of *Davidius moiwanus* (Gomphidae). Tombo, 16, 2–10.

Ballard, J. W. & Whitelock, M. C. (2004) The incomplete natural history of mitochondria. *Molecular Ecology*, 13, 729–744.

Bartenev, A. N. (1914) Materiaux pour lietude de la faune de Libellules de la Siberie, 16, 17. *Horae Societatis Entomologicae Rossicae*, 41, 1–32.

Brower, A. V. Z. (1994) Rapid morphological radiation and convergence among races of the butterfly *Heliconius erato* inferred from patterns of mitochondrial DNA evolution. *Proceedings of the National Academy of Sciences of the United States of America*, 91, 6491–6495.

Farrell, B. D. (2001) Evolutionary assembly of the milkweed fauna: cytocchrome oxidase I and the age of *Tetraopes* beetles. *Molecular Phylogenetics and Evolution*, 18, 467–478.

Funk, D. J. & Omland, K. E. (2003) Species-level paraphyly and polyphyly; frequency, causes, and consequences, with insights fromm animal mitochondrial DNA. *Annual Review of Ecology, Evolution and Systematics*, 34, 397–423.

Ichikawa, K., Fujita, Y. & Shimazu, M. (1970) The Geologic Development of the Japanese Islands. (in Japanese) Tokyo:Tsukiji-shokan.

Iijima, A. & Tada, R. (1990) Evolution and Tertiary sedimentary basins of Japan in reference to opening of the Japan Sea. Journal of the Faculty of Science, University of Tokyo. *Section II, Geology, mineralogy, geography, geophysics*, 22, 121–171.

Ishida, S., Ishida, K., Kojima, K & Sugimura, M. (1988). Illustrated guide for identification of the Japanese Odonata. Sapporo:Tokai University Press.

Kitamura, A., Takano, O., Takata, H. and Omote, H. (2001) Late Pliocene-early Pleistocene paleoceanographic evolution f the Sea of Japan. *Palaeogeography, Palaeoclimatology, Palaeoecology*, 172, 81–98.

Kiyoshi, T. (2008). Differentiation of golden-ringed dragonfly *Anotogaster sieboldii* (Selys, 1854) (Cordulegastridae: Odonata) in the insular East Asia revealed by the mitochondrial gene genealogy with taxonomic implications. *Journal of Zoological Systematics and Evolutionary Research*, 46, 105-109

Kiyoshi, T & Sota, T. (2006). Differentiation of the dragonfly genus *Davidius* (Odonata: Gomphidae) in Japan inferred from mitochondrial and nuclear gene genealogies. *Zoological Science*, 23, 1-8.

Kizaki, K. & Oshiro, I. (1980) The origin of the Ryukyu Island. In: Kizaki, K., (Ed). Natural History of the Ryukyu. (pp. 8–37) Tokyo: Tsukiji-Shokan. (in Japanese).

Machida, H., Ota, Y., Kawano, T., Moriwaki, H. & Nagaoka, S. (2001) Regional Geomorphology of the Japanese Islands, Vol. 7. Geomorphology of Kyushu and the Ryukyu. Tokyo: University of Tokyo Press. (in Japanese)

Odonatological Society of Osaka (1998) Dragonflies and Damselflies (Insecta: Odonata) of Shiga Prefecture, Honshu, Japan. *Research Report of the Lake Biwa Museum*, 10. (in Japanese).

Osawa, S., Su, Z. & Imura, Y. (2002) Molecular phylogeny and evolution of the carabid groud beetles of the World. Tokyo: Tetsugakushobo. (in Japanese)

Ota, H. (1998) Geographic patterns of endemism and speciation in amphibians and reptiles of the Ryukyu Archipelago, Japan, with special reference to their paleogeographical implications. *Researchs on Population Ecology*, 40, 189–204.

Quek, S. P., Davies, S. J., Itino, T. & Pierce, N. E. (2004) Codiversification in an ant-plant mutualism: stem texure and the evolution of host use in *Crematogaster* (Formicidae: Myrmicinae) inhabitants of *Macaranga* (Euphrbiaceae). *Evolution*, 58, 554–570.

Raymond, M. & Rousset, F. (1995) An exact test for population differentiation. *Evolution*, 58, 554–570.

Ryder, O. A. (1986) Species conservation and systematics: the dilemma of subspecies. *Trends in Ecology and Evoluiton*, 1, 9–10.

Sugimura, M., Ishida, S., Kojima, K., Ishida, K & Aoki, T. (1999). Dragonflies of the Japanese Archipelago in color. Sapporo: Hokkaido University Press.

Tada, R. (1994) Paleoceanographic evolution of the Japan Sea. *Palaeogeography Palaeoclimatology Palaeoecology*, 108: 487–508.

Tominaga, O., Su, Z. H., Kim, C. G., Okamoto, M., Imura, Y. & Osawa, S. (2000) Formation of the Japanese carabid fauna inferred from a phylogenetic tree of mitochondrial ND5 gene sequences (Coleoptera, Carabidae). *Journal of Molecular Evolution*, 50, 541–549

Tsuda, S. (2000). A distributional list of world Odonata 2000. Osaka: published by the author.

Wang, L. J. (2000) Dragonflies of Taiwan. Taipei: Jenjiem Calendar Co.

Watanabe, K., Takahashi, H., Kitamura, A., Yokoyama, R., Kitagawa, T., Takeshima, H., Sato, S., Yamamoto, S., Takehana, Y., Mukai, T., Ohara, K. & Iguchi, K. (2006) Biogeographical history of Japanese freshwater fishes: Phylogeographic approaches and perspectives. *Japanese Journal of Ichthyology*, 53, 1–38.

Wheeler, W. C. (1996) Optimization alignment: the end of multiple sequence alignment in phylogenetics?, *Cladistics*, 12, 1–9.

Yonekura, N., Kaizuka, S., Nogami, M. & Chinzei, K. (2001) Regional Geomorphology of the Japanese Islands, Vol. 1: Introduction to Japanese Geomorphology. Tokyo: University of Tokyo Press. (in Japanese)

Zhao, X. (1990) The gomphid dragonflies of China. (Odonata: Gomphidae). Fuzhou: The Science and Technology Publishing House.

In: Phylogeography
Editor: Damien S. Rutgers

ISBN: 978-1-60692-954-4
© 2013 Nova Science Publishers, Inc.

Chapter 7

Statistical Phylogeography, Ecological Niche Models and Predicting Glacial Refugia: An Examination of Key Assumptions

Nathan G. Swenson[1] and Jason Pither[2]

[1] Center for Tropical Forest Science – Asia Program
Arnold Arboretum Harvard University
Cambridge, Massachusetts, US
[2] Biology and Physical Geography
University of British Columbia Okanagan
Kelowna, British Columbia, Canada

Abstract

Recent statistical phylogeographic work has sought to integrate ecological niche models (ENMs) into phylogeography as a methodology for testing and formulating hypotheses regarding the geographic histories of species. The lure of ENMs lies in their ability to use present day climatic and physiographic affinities of species to predict the past geographic distributions of these same species under different climatic regimes. These predicted distributions can then be used to evaluate the likelihood and location of glacial refugia. Given the bourgeoning interest in ENMs, now is an appropriate time for phylogeographers to reexamine their conceptual and methodological foundations. We argue that in the rush to assimilate this methodology, critical underlying assumptions have not been adequately considered. Here we discuss some of the fundamental assumptions underlying ENMs and how their violation may lead to faulty phylogeographic inferences. We will conclude by discussing alternative avenues for future research that will enable a more reliable and fruitful integration of ENM and phylogeography.

[1] Email: nswenson@oeb.harvard.edu
[2] Email: jason.pither@ubc.ca

ECOLOGICAL NICHE MODELS AND PHYLOGEOGRAPHY

Ecological niche models (ENMs) generally use the observed correlation between species occurrence and abiotic variables to predict the present day, past or future geographic range of the species of interest. The reader is directed to Elith et al. 2006 for a thorough review of ENMs. The potential power of this approach and the ease with which it can be applied are obvious and the usage of ENMs has spread in ecology and evolution at an impressive rate (Elith et al. 2006; Swenson 2008). Recently, evolutionary biologists in general, and phylogeographers in particular, have begun to incorporate ENMs into their research (Hugall et al. 2002; Graham et al. 2004; Kidd and Ritchie 2006; Carstens and Richards 2007; Richards et al. 2007; Swenson 2008). While ecologists have generally focused on predicting the extent of species in the present and in the future, phylogeographers have been more interested in predicting the past distribution of species or populations. In particular, phylogeographers have been interested in using ENMs to determine whether species or populations were constrained to refugia during periods of glacial advance. Because ENMs only need present day species occurrence data and estimated maps of past climates, phylogeographers are able to quickly apply this method to address some of the long-standing questions regarding the influence of climatic oscillations and concurrent range contraction into glacial refugia in producing lineage diversification. Thus, the interest in incorporating ENMs into the analytical toolkit used by phylogeographers is obvious. That said, we believe that in the rush to incorporate ENMs into phylogeography, phylogeographers have failed to adequately appreciate the myriad of assumptions associated with ENMs, and to fully consider how the violation of these assumptions affects phylogenetic inferences. Here, we outline what we consider to be several critical assumptions underlying ENMs. We briefly discuss why each assumption is likely to be violated in practice, and describe example consequences of such violations. We conclude with a statement concerning alternative pathways towards the integration of ENMs and phylogeography.

ASSUMPTIONS AND REASON FOR CONCERN

In this section we outline five implicit or explicit assumptions associated with ENMs that we believe are critical in determining the quality of the inferences that they provide. We acknowledge that there are a number of other assumptions that we do not highlight that are also important for the user to consider (e.g. the importance of interactions among trophic levels).

Assumption 1: The Abiotic Control Assumption

The influences of biotic interactions (and specifically, competition) on species' contemporary distributions are negligible relative to the influences of the environment. This assumption ultimately stems from traditional perspectives of the niche (Hutchinson 1957; Whittaker 1975), and more specifically, the idea that species' fundamental environmental optima (i.e. the abiotic conditions under which species achieve maximum performance) have evolved to be distinct from one-another, thanks to past competitive interactions fostering niche divergence (Whittaker 1975). In other words, by assuming that competition in the past fostered niche divergence among species, one sets the stage for the argument that species' contemporary distributions are governed primarily by the environment, and only minimally by biotic interactions. However, a variety of ecological, biogeographic, and evolutionary processes could lead to co-distributed species having effectively equivalent fundamental environmental niches (including optima) as opposed to distinct ones (Leibold and McPeek, 2006), in which case we should expect species' realized distributions (and thus realized niches) to reflect the vagaries of competitive interactions in addition to species-environment matching. For example, plants are thought to conform to dominance-tolerance hierarchies (also called a "shared preferences" model of fundamental niche differentiation; Rosenzweig 1991; Wisheu, 1998), whereby tolerators with broad fundamental niches share similar optima with environmental specialists, but are competitively excluded from optimal environments by the specialists. Under this scenario, the accuracy of ENMs that are used to predict historical or future distributions will depend critically upon the "competitive milieu" being identical to the one that informed the model (see Assumption 2). If, for example, the specialist species was historically absent from the regions of interest, then the tolerator species would likely have occupied a very different range compared to what the ENM would predict (it would have occupied more optimal environments). This could lead to ENMs predicting the occurrence of glacial refugia where in reality there were none (Swenson 2008). In summary, the validity of the 'abiotic control' assumption depends critically upon species having evolved divergent fundamental environmental optima; yet, this scenario of fundamental niche differentiation is no more likely than any other, including ones that include prevalent niche equivalence (e.g. Leibold and McPeek, 2006),   ENM predictions should therefore be carefully considered in the light of multiple, alternative scenarios of fundamental niche differentiation.

Assumption 2: Communities Are Closed Systems Through Space and Time

ENMs are generally only parameterized using abiotic correlative relationships. As such, they implicitly assume either that biotic interactions do not matter (see assumption 1), or that they do matter but are invariant in space and time. On the contrary, it is widely accepted that communities are not closed systems (Gleason 1926; Leibold et al. 2004,) and biotic interactions including competition are thought to influence the distributions of species (MacArthur 1972; Gaston, 2003). Furthermore, species are expected to engage in novel interactions as their distributions shift with changing climates (Harrington et al. 1999). These novel interactions may facilitate or retard the range extension or contraction of species. Thus, it is not possible to determine whether ENMs are likely to over- or under-predict the ranges of species because the novel and pre-existing biotic interactions that help shape the distribution of that species are not considered.

Assumption 3: Historical Climate Data are Accurate and Non-Analog Climates are Unimportant

Phylogeographers using ENMs to predict the historical distribution of species must rely on historical climate predictions being accurate. In ENM studies that predict the historical distribution of species it is assumed that the climatic predictions are robust and that species responses to non-analog climates can be predicted based on present day climates. The quality of the different historical climate predictions is difficult to determine, but will surely vary in quality geographically and temporally. For example, regions of high topographic relief are likely to be associated with higher uncertainty in climate predictions, yet these same regions are often among the most interesting from a phylogeographic perspective (e.g. Carstens and Richards 2007). In any case, we argue that uncertainties in historical climate predictions should be explicitly discussed within phylogeographic studies. Our first point here is not diminish the historical climate estimates that have been made; rather we simply note that ENM users generally treat these climate estimates as fixed values that lack error, when clearly this is not the case. Our second concern regards the ability to predict the response of species to non-analog climates based on their response to present day conditions. Non-analog climates are unique combinations of singular climate axes, which produce a completely novel multidimensional climate (Jackson and Williams, Frontiers in Ecology paper, 2008?). ENMs consider the correlation between present day species occurrences and one to several climatic axes. Even if ENMs do consider multiple climatic axes at once they will never, by definition, have data relating species to non-analog climates. Thus the species may be (i) predicted to be absent from non-analog climates by an ENM because that climate does not presently exist, or (ii) it is predicted to be present in non-analog climates by an ENM because it occupies a modern analog that is somewhat, but not entirely, similar. We argue that both of these outcomes are at best uninformative, or worse, misleading. Recent work has shown that non-analog climates are a frequent occurrence as the climate changes and that it is often hard to predict how species will respond to these novel climates (Jackson and Overpeck 2000; Williams et al. 2007). Thus, we consider it highly likely that the assumption that species responses to non-analog climates are unimportant or that they can be predicted from current day species distributions is often violated.

Assumption 4: Landmass Dynamics Are Known or Static

In order to predict the historical range of a species with an ENM, the researcher needs a map of the historical climate and the historical physiography. In most cases to date the historical physiography has been considered constant. That is, the topography and size of landmasses have not changed. Because the majority of phylogeographic studies that have used ENMs have projected the distribution of species during the Pleistocene glaciation, it seems reasonable to assume that the topography of the study region has not changed too greatly. On the other hand, the sizes of landmasses and the positioning of coastlines have not been static. During glaciation the sea level is substantially reduced and the available landmass is generally greatly expanded. Thus, it is simply inappropriate to predict the Pleistocene distribution of species using present day coastlines. The lower Pleistocene sea levels in many cases may have promoted the dispersal of organisms within and between landmasses and by not incorporating this reality into ENMs, they may predict overly constrained historical distributions of species. A similar caution relates to inland water bodies, as these are likely to have played a critical role in the historical dynamics of many species.

Assumption 5: Critical Abiotic Variables are Known

The success of ENMs, or generally any model, critically relies upon the quality of the data used to generate it. The user of ENMs generates the predicted range using the known current location of the species and the underlying environment at those locations. In most cases that researcher will utilize a set of commonly used 'bioclimatic variables' to represent the underlying environment (I.E. http://www.worldclim.org/). While species likely do respond differentially to these bioclimatic variables, it is likely that in many cases the critical variable limiting the distribution of the species of interest in not represented in this generic list of bioclimatic variables. Thus, models that lack the critical limiting variable are likely to produce poor predictions. One might argue that this problem is avoided if the critical variable co-varies strongly and predictably with one of the included variables. However, relying on proxy variables is risky, because they are unlikely to exhibit a straightforward relationship to the limiting variable under all situations. In short, there is often no *a priori* reasoning by the researcher for why he or she is using certain bioclimatic variables in an ENM. We argue that ENM users should first either consult the physiological ecology literature pertaining to the species they wish to study or perform physiological tolerance experiments to determine what are the key variables that limit the performance of their organism and then use those variables to construct their ENMs.

CONCLUSION

The field of phylogeography has begun to embrace the enticing range predictions generated by ENMs. In the rush to incorporate this technology into phylogeography, we fear that phylogeographers will not consider some of the critical implicit and explicit assumptions that ENMs make. In this commentary, we have outlined several of these assumptions followed by brief arguments for not only how they are likely violated, but also how this might severely reduce the quality of the inferences made in ENM research.

Despite our cautionary notes, we are not against the application of ENMs in phylogeography. Rather we think that the above assumptions should be more carefully considered and that a new generation of ENMs could be constructed that will strengthen our inferences. We hope that this next generation of ENMs would take a more physiological approach where models are parameterized based upon the physiological performance and the population biology (Buckley 2008; Swenson 2008; Kearney and Porter 2009) of the organisms in different environments. We also feel that there should be a concurrent focus on the abiotic and biotic environment in ENM algorithms allowing for the entire ecological context to be modeled. If these initial obstacles can be overcome we feel that ENMs may be of greater to use in the field of phylogeography, but until that time a greater appreciation of the assumptions involved with currently implemented ENMs is required.

ACKNOWLEDGMENTS

NGS was supported by a NSF Post-Doctoral Fellowship in Bioinformatics. JP is supported by a NSERC Discovery Grant (Canada), and a UBC Okanagan start-up grant. Both authors have benefitted from conversations with Michael Weiser on this topic.

REFERENCES

Buckley, L.B. 2008. Linking traits to energetics and population dynamics to predict lizard ranges in changing environments. *American Naturalist* 171:E1-E19.

Carstens, B.C., and C.L. Richards. 2007. Integrating coalescent and ecological niche modeling in comparative phylogeography. *Evolution* 61:1439-1454.

Elith, J., C.H. Graham, R.P. Anderson, M. Dudyk, S. Ferrier, A. Guisan, R.J. Hijmans, F. Huettmann, J.R. Leathwick, A. Lehmann, J. Li, L.G. Lohmann, B.A. Loiselle, G. Manion, C. Moritz, M. Nakamura, Y. Nakazawa, J.M. Overton, A.T. Peterson, S.J. Phillips, K. Richardson, R. Scachetti-Pereira, R.E. Schapire, J. Soberon, S. Williams, M.S. Wisz, and N.E. Zimmermann, N.E. 2006. Novel methods improve prediction of species' distributions from occurrence data. *Ecography* 29:129–151.

Gaston, K. J. 2003. The structure and dynamics of geographic ranges. Oxford University Press, New York.

Gleason, H.A. 1926. The individualist concept of the plant association. *Bulletin of the Torrey Botanical Club* 53:7-26.

Graham, C.H., R.R. Santiago, J.C. Santos, C.J. Schneider, and C. Moritz. 2004. Integrating phylogenetics and environmental niche models to explore speciation mechanisms in Dendrobatid frogs. *Evolution* 58:1781-1793.

Harrington, R., I Woiwod, and T. Sparks. 1999. Climate change and trophic interactions. *Trends in Ecology and Evolution* 14:146-150.

Hugall, A., C. Moritz, A. Moussalli, and J. Stanisic. 2002. Reconciling paleodistribution models and comparative phylogeography in the Wet Tropics rainforest land snail *Gnarosophia bellendenkerensis* (Brazier 1875) *Proceedings of the National Academy of Sciences U.S.A.* 99:6112-6117

Hutchinson, G.E. 1957. Concluding remarks. *Cold Spring Harbor Symposium on Quantitative Biology* 22:415-427.

Jackson, S.T., and J.T. Overpeck. 2000. Responses of plant populations and communities to environmental changes of the Late Quaternary. *Paleobiology* 26:S194-S220.

Kearney, M., and W. Porter. 2009. Mechanistic range modeling: combining physiological and spatial data to predict species' ranges. *Ecology Letters* 12:334-350.

Kidd, D. M., and M. G. Ritchie. 2006. Phylogeographic information systems; Putting the geography into phylogeography. *Journal of Biogeography* 33:1851-1865.

Leibold, M. A., M. Holyoak, N. Mouquet, P. Amarasekare, J. M. Chase, M. F. Hoopes, R. D. Holt, J. B. Shurin, R. Law, D. Tilman, M. Loreau, and A. Gonzalez. 2004. The metacommunity concept: a framework for multi-scale community ecology. *Ecology Letters*, 7:601-613.

Leibold, M.A. and McPeek, M.A. 2006. Coexistence of the niche and neutral perspectives in community ecology. *Ecology*, 87:1399-1410.

MacArthur, R.H. 1972. *Geographical Ecology: Patterns in the Distribution of Species.* Harper and Row.

MacArthur, M.L. 1995. *Species Diversity in Space and Time.* Cambridge University Press, Cambridge.

Richards, C.L., B.C. Carstens, and L.L. Knowles. 2007. Distribution modeling and statistical phylogeography: An integrative framework for generating and testing alternative biogeographic hypotheses. *Journal of Biogeography* 34:1833-1845.

Rosenzweig, M. L. 1991. Habitat selection and population interactions: the search for mechanism. *American Naturalist*, 137:S5-S28.

Swenson, N.G. 2008. The past and future influence of geographic information systems on hybrid zone, phylogeographic and speciation research. *Journal Evolutionary Biology* 21:421-434.

Whittaker, R.H. 1975. *Communities and Ecosystems.* New York, New York.

Williams, J.W., S.T. Jackson, and J.E. Kutzbach. 2007. Projecting distributions of novel and disappearing climates by 2100 AD. *Proceedings of the National Academy of Sciences U.S.A.* 104:5738-5742.

Wisheu, I. C. 1998. How organisms partition habitats: different types of community organization can produce identical patterns. *Oikos,* 83:246-258.

In: Phylogeography
Editor: Damien S. Rutgers

ISBN: 978-1-60692-954-4
© 2013 Nova Science Publishers, Inc.

Chapter 8

THE NEED FOR A MULTISPECIES, MULTILOCUS PHYLOGEOGRAPHICAL APPROACH

*Cristiano Vernesi**

Centro di Ecologia Alpina – Research and Innovation Centre, Fondazione Edmund Mach
Viote del Monte Bondone, Trento, Italy

INTRODUCTION

Phylogeography (Avise et al, 1987) focuses on the study of the geographical structure of gene lineages within single species. The aim to analyze how phylogenetic relationships of genealogical lineages are distributed across the geographical landscape makes phylogeography a discipline embedded in the wider field of biogeography which is primarily concerned with inference and, possibly, identification of the major processes shaping organismal diversity at different levels of geographical and taxonomical scales.

The adoption of molecular data to infer patterns of genetic variation interpreted in a geographical context positively affected biogeographical research: many fruitful insights can be gained about the different roles of bottlenecks, population expansions, vicariance and gene flow in structuring genetic variability (Avise, 2000, Knowles and Maddison, 2002).

From its inception, at least two major breakthroughs occurred in phylogeography: the advent of comparative phylogeography (Cracraft, 1989; Riddle, 1996; Zink, 1996) and the use of model-based statistical analysis which led to statistical phylogeography (Knowles and Maddison, 2002; Knowles, 2004; Knowles, 2008).

The comparative approach involves the comparison among co-distributed taxa of geographical patterns of genetic variation thus allowing detailed inferences to be drawn about, for instance, landscape evolution, dispersal across a region, speciation, extinction and adaptive radiation. Linking population processes to regional biogeographical and diversity patterns can have important outcomes also for ecology and evolution studies (Bermingham and Moritz, 1998). Historically and evolutionary independent regions can be identified, statistically testing their independence through adequate state-of-art analytical methods.

---

* E-mail: vernesi@cealp.it

Determining the evolutionary and geographical framework, phlyogeography can shed light on the spatial and historical influences governing the distribution of species richness in ecological communities (Ricklefs and Schluter, 1993). Finally, the possibility to identify evolutionary isolated areas is of great importance as a tool to better design conservation strategies (Moritz and Faith, 1998).

The efforts to preserve and manage biodiversity can, therefore, greatly benefit from the results of comparative phylogeography by allowing understanding the processes responsible, both locally and a regional level, for origin, evolution, diversification and maintenance of communities (Bermingham and Moritz, 1998).

The advent of several coalescent-based analytical methods has somehow revolutionized the interpretation of genetic data; instead of simply describing the data in search of *ad hoc* explanations, it's now possible to statistically test whether the data fit some historical and demographic scenario (Knowles and Maddison, 2002). Several hypotheses about the processes underlying patterns of genetic variability and structure can now rigorously tested in a reasonable amount of computation time, thanks also to the technical improvement in computer technology.

It is now widely recognized that further development of coalescent-based methods, also with extensive use of Bayesian approaches, can significantly contribute to phylogeography studies (Avise, 2009).

Despite these premises, it seems that most of current phylogeographical literature is still centered around the analysis of a single genetic marker in a single species.

SINGLE VS MULTIPLE LOCI ISSUE

As we noted, an increasing number of phlyogeography studies relies on coalescent-based methods for estimating several relevant population parameters such as effective population size, migration rate, divergence time, growth rate, time elapsed since the onset of a demographic expansion.

It is well known from population genetics theory that the stochastic nature of the genealogical process implies a considerable amount of variance associated with parameters estimation (see e.g. Wakeley, 2008). However, it is also known that variance associated with coalescent estimates can be significantly reduced increasing the number of independent loci analyzed (Pluzhnikov and Donnelly, 1996). While the genealogy of such loci are independent, that is they can be seen as random draws from the distribution over all possible genealogies, the distribution will ultimately depend on the demographic history of the population.

Thus, our phylogeographic interest in inferring population history by means of molecular data should be regularly based on multiple loci. Pursuing this approach nonetheless harbors its specific problems: the independent nuclear loci employed usually have low mutation rates, especially when compared to mitochondrial markers. However, each single incompletely resolved nuclear gene tree, when summed over multiple loci, provides enough signal for inference (Hare et al, 2002). Among-locus variation in mutation rate is another well recognized source of bias in coalescent estimates (Takahata and Satta, 1997; Yang, 1997): it seems that insofar multilocus studies recorded among-locus rate variation sufficiently low to not severely affect parameters estimates (Yang, 2002; Wall, 2003; Jennings and Edwards, 2005). A third major drawback is represented by recombination at both intra- and inter-locus level. Also in this case, nonetheless, some useful precautions can be adopted: analyzing different data partitions separately would greatly reduce the risk of intralocus recombination (Hare, 2001; Hugall et al, 2002) while choosing markers located on separate chromosome would strongly decrease the probability of inter locus recombination. It is worth noting that, at any rate, recombination events can be effectively incorporated in coalescent models (Wakeley, 2008).

With several independent loci, the problem arises how to interpret the different gene genealogies. The solution can simply be based upon the assumption that the demographic history of a population leaves signature at the genome level, thus affecting most of the loci analyzed. In contrast, selection is expected to act on single markers, according to the adaptive trait, directly or indirectly, controlled by the marker itself. This line of reasoning formed the basis of the classical approach by Lewontin and Krakauer (1973) for testing selective neutrality: while most of neutral markers reflect population history and are, therefore, expected to record similar amount of genetic differentiation as measured with Fst, loci under some selective constraints would display 'outlier' Fst values. After some decades, the so called Fst outlier method was re-discovered with development of specific statistical methods (Beaumont and Nichols, 1996; Vitalis et al, 2001; Beaumont and Balding, 2004).

Under a gene genealogy perspective, the wide spectrum of topology that can arise from stochastic sorting of independent genes among different lineages (Avise and Wollenberg, 1997) makes it untenable to derive conclusions from the simple visual interpretation of the genealogies. But, it is indeed the among-locus variation in coalescence patterns that can be adequately exploited in estimating population parameters (Edwards and Beerli, 2000; Dolman and Moritz, 2006; Carstens and Knowles, 2007). In this case use of specific multilocus coalescent models (e.g. Hey and Nielsen, 2004) allows retrieving crucial information for inferring historical demography. While these methods usually entail a non negligible amount of uncertainty in parameters estimation, typically exemplified by large confidence intervals, such uncertainty can be significantly reduced analyzing a number of loci in the order to about five to ten. While almost impossible just few years ago, these numbers are now achievable in most non-model organisms due to impressive improvement in sequencing technologies (Shendure and Ji, 2008) and concomitant reduction in costs (Schloss, 2008).

THE IMPORTANCE OF GEOGRAPHY

Reviewing the recent phylogeography literature is quite evident that most of the studies are predominantly centered around a species or a complex of closely-related species. As noted by Kidd and Ritchie (2006), the geographical component seems in minority in comparison to the 'phylo' component. These authors placed particular emphasis on the need to better integrate GIS-based techniques with genetic-based data. In our opinion it is not only a matter of methodological tools, yet of the utmost importance. What phylogeography seems too often to neglect, it is a clear focus on a particular area (or better ecosystem), preferring, as starting point, to focus on a particular species. Of course, inference of historical and evolutionary patterns acting on a species are of vital importance but none of us would deny that the current biodiversity crisis prompts for actions on a wider scale (Wilson et al, 2007; Pressey et al, 2007). Challenges posed by global change require that all scientific disciplines devoted to understanding processes of biological diversity concentrate their efforts at the ecosystem level. It is now becoming more evident that genetic variation in one species can promote ecological consequences to the entire community (Johnson and Stinchcombe, 2007).

The possibility of a cross-contamination among methodological approaches usually set apart, such as those of spatial ecology and phylogeography, can have profound impacts in analyzing patterns and elucidating processes of genetic variability and structure referred not just to a single species but to an entire particular area. Ecological niche models, paleodistribution models and coalescent-based simulation proved very useful to this end (Hugall et al, 2002; Knowles et al, 2007; Richards et al 2007.

SYNTHESIS

Our impression is that the time has come for phylogeography to move a step forward, trying to integrate the most notable advancements of the last years, the comparative approach and the extensive use of multilocus coalescent-based models.

Obviously it is not just a matter of studying patterns of genetic variability and structure in a random pick of species inhabiting a more or less restricted geographic area. Some kind of rationale should inform the selection of the species, also for avoiding the risk of over interpreting the data in the search of a common pattern.

Unfortunately, it is absolutely not an easy task to accomplish the identification of the most relevant species expected to play a central role in a community. Most of the research insofar performed seems to have been based on theoretical background (see e.g. Ebenmann and Jonsson, 2005; Vellend, 2006) with scarce empirical applications (for a review see Randall Hughes et al, 2008).

We strongly believe that the selection of the species should be based on some form of ecological considerations (trophic interaction, complementarity of roles, etc.): for this reason, it would be highly desirable a tighter interaction between ecologists and phylogeographers. Not only the species would be selected more adequately but also the sampling scheme could greatly benefit from such an interplay.

It is clear that this integrated approach is far from being easily affordable, but, at the same time, the complexity of the challenges posed to biodiversity by multifaceted effects of global change urgently calls for new approaches to be explored.

Retrieval of historical demography and evolutionary parameters across different species of the same area would immediately allow inferring processes acting on a geographic scale from those species-specific. Testing of biogeographical scenarios would be more robust if we could, not only qualitatively, assess different hypotheses in a set of ecologically related species. Areas of particular evolutionary relevance would be identified, also in light of more informed management and conservation strategies. We now realize that biodiversity conservation policies are more effective when centered around a specific, yet relatively restricted area, than to just some iconic or charismatic species.

The striking advancement in sequencing technology makes it possible not only to think at the simultaneous analysis of several loci but also to cost effectively pursue this task, even in non-model organisms, like those usually addressed by most phylogeographical studies. In some sense, it has to be admitted that phylogeography too has to enter the (post) genomic era. We argue that a shift from single to multilocus analysis should be accompanied by the concomitant shift from a single to multi-species approach. Further, since our interest is mainly about the inference of past patterns and processes, this approach would gain further strength including analysis of historical and museum DNA. Also in this latter case, the technology advancement might play a significant role.

To conclude, it seems that the track has already been traced through the recent improvements in the phylogeography field: analysis of multiple loci across a set of ecologically relevant species. Now it's time to move along this track with the ultimate goal of contributing to better understand and preserve organismal diversity at both regional and local scale.

REFERENCES

Avise JC, (2004). Molecular Markers, Natural History, and Evolution. Sunderland, Massachusetts, USA, Sinauer Associates, Inc. Publishers.

Avise JC, (2009). Phylogeography: retrospect and prospect. *Journal of Biogeography*, 3-15.

Avise JC, Arnold J, Ball RM, Bermingham E, Lamb T, Neigl JE, Reeb CA, Saunders NC (1987). The mitochondrial DNA bridge between populations genetics and systematics. *Annual Review of Ecology and Systematics,* 457.498.

Avise JC, Wollenberg K, (1997). Phylogenetics and the oiigin of species. *Proc. Natl. Acad. Sci. USA*, 7748-7755.

Beaumont MA, Balding DJ, (2004). Identifying adaptive genetic divergence among populations from genome scans. *Molecular Ecology*, 969-980.

Beaumont MA, Nichols RA, (1996). Evaluating loci for use in the gnetic analysis of population structure. *Proceedings of the Royal Society of London Series*, 1619-1626.

Bermingham E, Moritz C. (1998). Comparative phylogeography: concepts and applications. *Molecular Ecology*, 367-369.

Carstens BC, Knowles LL, (2007). Shifting distributions and speciation: genomic resolution of species divergence during rapid climate change. *Molecular Ecology*, 619-627.

Cracraft J, (1989). Speciation and its ontology: the empirical consequences of alternative specis concepts for understanding patterns and proceses of differentiation. *Speciation and its consequences*, 28-59.

Dolman G, Moritiz C, (2006). A multilocus perspective on refugial isolation and divergence in rainforest skinks. *Evolution*, (Carlia), 573-582.

Edwards SV, Beerli, P, (2000). Perspective: gene divergence and population divergence, and the variance in coalescence time in phylogeographic studies. *Evolution*, 1839-1854.

Hare MP, Cipriano F, Palumbi (2002). Genetic evidence on the demography of speciation in allopatric dolphin species. *Evolution*, 804-816.

Hare P, (2001). Prospects for nuclear gene phylogeography. *Trends in Ecology and Evolution*, 700-706.

Hey J, Nielsen R, (2004). Multilocus methods for estimating population sizes, migration rates and divergence time, with applications to the divergence of Drospohila pseudoobscura and D. persimilis. *Genetics*, 747-760.

Jennings WB, Edwards SV, (2005). Speciational history of Australian grass finches (Poephila) inferred from thirty gene trees. *Evolution*, 2033-2047.

Kidd DM, Ritchie MG1461462006N146146 Phylogeographic information systems: putting the geography into phylogeography. *Journal of Biogeography*, 1851-1865.

Knowles LL, (2004). The burgeoning field of statistical phylogeography. *Journal of Evolutionary Biology*, 1-10.

Knowles LL, (2008). Statistical phylogeography: the use of coalescent approaches to infer evoltionary history. *Annual Review of Ecology, Evolution, and Systematics*, in press.

Knowles LL, Maddison WP (2002). Statistical phylogeography. *Molecular Ecology*, 2623-2635.

Lewontin RC, Krakauer J, (1973). Distribution of gene frequency as a test of the theory of selective neutrality of polymorphisms. *Genetics*, 175-195.

Moritz C, Faith DP (1998). Comparative phylogeography and the identification of genetically divergent areas for conservation. *Molecular Ecology*, 419-429.

Otte D, Endler JA and Sunderland, MA, USA, Sinauer Inc. Publishers.

Pluzhnikov A, Donnelly P, (1996). Optimal sequencing strategies for surveying molecular genetic diversity. *Genetics*, 1247-1262.

Pressey RL, Cabeza M, Watts M, Cowling RM, Wilson K, (2007). Conservation planning in a changing world. *Trends in Ecology and Evolution*, 583-592.

Richards CL, Carstens BC, Knowles LL, (2007). Distribution model and statistical phylogeography: an integrative framework for generating and testing alternative biogeographical hypotheses. *Journal of Biogeography*, 1833-1845.

Ricklefs RE, Schluter D. (1993). Species Diversity in Ecological Communities: Historical and Geographical Perspectives. Chicago, IL, USA, University of Chicago Press.

Riddle BR, (1996). The molecular phylogeographic bridge between deep and shallow history in continental biotas. *Trends in Ecology and Evolution*, 207-211.

Schloss JA, (2008). How to get genomes at one ten-thousandth the cost. *Nature Biotechnology*, 1113-1115.

Shendure J, Ji H, (2008). Next-generation DNA sequencing. *Nature Biotechnology*, 1135-1145.

Takahata N, Satta Y, (1997). Evolution of the primate lineage leading to modern humans: phylogenetic and demographic inferences from DNA sequence data. *Proc. Natl. Acad. Sci. USA*, 4811-4815.

Vitalis R, Dawson K, Boursot P, (2001). Interpretation of variation across marker loci as evidence of selection. *Genetics*, 1811-1823.

Wakeley J, (2008). Coalescent theory: an introduction Greenwood Village, Colorado, USA, Roberts & Company Publishers.

Wall JD, (2003). Estimating ancestral population sizes and divergence times. *Genetics*, 395-404.

Wilson KA, Underwood EC, Morrison SA, Klausmeyer KR, Murdoch WW, et al. (2007). Conserving Biodiversity Efficiently: What to Do, Where, and When 223.

Yang Z, (1997). On the estimation of ancestral population sizes of modern humans. *Genet. Res. Camb.* 11-116.

Yang Z, (2002). Likelihood and bayes estimation of ancestral population sizes in hominoids using data from multiple loci. *Genetics*, 1811-1823.

Zink RM, (1996). Comparative phylogeography of North America birds. *Evolution*, 307-318.

In: Phylogeography
Editor: Damien S. Rutgers

Chapter 9

PHYLOGEOGRAPHY OF FINCHES AND SPARROWS[*]

Antonio Arnaiz-Villena[†], Pablo Gomez-Prieto
and Valentin Ruiz-del-Valle
Department of Immunology, University Complutense,
the Madrid Regional Blood Center, Madrid, Spain

ABSTRACT

Fringillidae finches form a subfamily of songbirds (*Passeriformes*), which are presently distributed around the world. This subfamily includes canaries, goldfinches, greenfinches, rosefinches, and grosbeaks, among others. Molecular phylogenies obtained with mitochondrial DNA sequences show that these groups of finches are put together, but with some polytomies that have apparently evolved or radiated in parallel. The time of appearance on Earth of all studied groups is suggested to start after Middle Miocene Epoch, around 10 million years ago.

Greenfinches (genus *Carduelis*) may have originated at Eurasian desert margins coming from *Rhodopechys obsoleta* (dessert finch) or an extinct pale plumage ancestor; it later acquired green plumage suitable for the greenfinch ecological niche, i.e.: woods. Multicolored Eurasian goldfinch (*Carduelis carduelis*) has a genetic extant ancestor, the green-feathered *Carduelis citrinella* (citril finch); this was thought to be a canary on phonotypical bases, but it is now included within goldfinches by our molecular genetics phylograms. Speciation events between citril finch and Eurasian goldfinch are related with the Mediterranean Messinian salinity crisis (5 million years ago). *Linurgus olivaceus* (oriole finch) is presently thriving in Equatorial Africa and was included in a separate genus (*Linurgus*) by itself on phenotypical bases. Our phylograms demonstrate that it is and old canary.

Proposed genus *Acanthis* does not exist. Twite and linnet form a separate radiation from redpolls. *Loxia* (crossbills) is an evolutive radiation which includes redpolls also. In

---

[*] A version of this chapter also appears in *Animal Genetics*, edited by Leopold J. Rechi, published by Nova Science Publishers, Inc. It was submitted for appropriate modifications in an effort to encourage wider dissemination of research.

[†] Corresponding author: Departamento de Inmunología, Facultad de Medicina, Universidad Complutense de Madrid, Avenida Complutense s/n, 28040 Madrid, Spain. Phone: +34 913017354; Fax: +34 913017356; E-mail address: aarnaiz@med.ucm.es; URL: http://chopo.pntic.mec.es/biolmol.

North America, three *Carduelis* radiations are found all coming from the Eurasian siskin: 1) that of American goldfinch, 2) the pine siskin one, and 3) the *Carduelis notata* one, ancestor of all South American siskins.

A new group of 'arid-zone' finches is genetically described that includes *Leucosticte arctoa*, *Carpodacus nipalensis*, *Rhodopechys githaginea* and *Rhodopechys mongolica*, at least.

Genus *Rhodopechys* should be redefined.

Pinicola enucleator (pine grosbeak) is the ancestor of bullfinches (genus *Pyrrhula*), forming a single evolutive radiation. Genus *Carpodacus* has been split in several evolutive radiations; American *Carpodacus* form a distinct evolution from Old World *Carpodacus*. *Haematospiza sipahi* is not a single genus, but a radiation together with *Carpodacus erythrinus*. Another evolutive radiation is found: *Uragus sibiricus* (a single species genus) radiated together with *Carpodacus rubicilloides*.

The grosbeak radiation (*Emberizinae*) occurred earlier than that of other *Fringillidae* birds and comprises genera *Coccothraustes*, *Eophona*, and *Mycerobas*. It is not discarded that New World grosbeaks (*Hesperiphona*) is also related.

Old World sparrows (genus *Passer*) conforms a single radiation starting in Africa (with *P. melanurus* and grey-headed sparrows), separated from *Ploceinae* and New and Old World *Emberizinae*. The closest radiation to genus *Passer* is genus *Petronia* (rock sparrows). *Passer hispaniolensis italiae* (brown head) is genetically closer to *P. domesticus* (grey head) than to *P. hispaniolensis* (brown head).

Subfamily Estrildinae cover a variety of finches widespread through Africa, Asia, Australia, and Indian and Pacific Ocean islands. Yet, many evolutive radiations are observed within this monophyletic group; they comprise birds from different continents: genetics does not correlate with geography in these birds. A possible origin for them is India since the basal and most ancient evolutive radiation —comprising African silverbill, Indian silverbill and (Australian) diamond firetail— may have started in India.

A clear example of convergent evolution is the case of American Carduelis dominicensis and African Linurgus olivaceus, which are very similar and acquire black head and greenish / yellow plumage in equatorial forests. Another fine example of phenotypic adaptation to environment is that of Serinus alario, the one black and white canary, because it nests on land or land / rocks. Finally, Eurasian goldfinch ancestor, mainly-green Carduelis citrinella, shows how plumage can change in relatively short times, as postulated.

In summary, some examples of evolution details and misclassification of songbirds are shown and put in a paleoclimatic and geographical context. This is now possible because of the existence of powerful computation methodologies for constructing molecular phylogenetic trees which are changing both our view of evolution and classification of living beings.

INTRODUCTION

It is admitted that present day bird species are originated from dinosaurs, with *Tyrannosaurus* having common ancestors with the present day birds (*Neornithes*). Apparently, radiation of these birds started to occur about 65 million years ago (MYA), in the Cretacic / Tertiary boundary [1].

Their crisis due to a meteorite impact and/or Indian subcontinent great volcano eruptions and other facts, led to the disappearance of many dinosaurs, but not all, like present day birds (*Neornithes*). Also, mammals, lizards, crocodiles, etc. passed through this 65 MYA extinction. Both, mammals and dinosaurs, appeared during Triassic age about 200 MYA, and have thrived until present times [1].

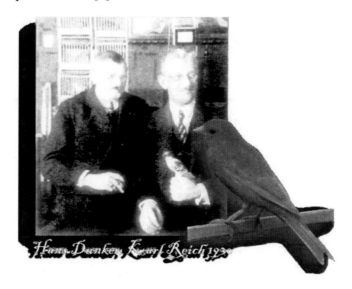

Figure 1. The red canary and its creators [4].

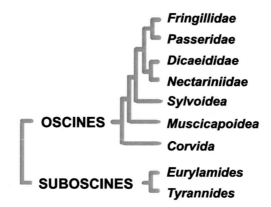

Figure 2. Proposed phylogenetic positioning of songbirds [3].

Mammals show now about 4200 different species and birds about 9600. However, it is possible that disappearance of terrestrial dinosaurs led to rapid occupation by mammals of some of the terrestrial ecological niches that had been left empty.

In the last 1500 years or so, 20% of dinosaur (bird) species have extinguished, 12% are now in great disappearance danger and most species are drastically decreasing number of individuals. This is all due to direct or indirect man activities [1,2].

About half of bird species belong to order *Passeriformes*, also known as 'songbirds' (Figure 2) [3]. This is divided into two suborders: *Passeri* (oscines) and *Tyranni* (suboscines, or New World *Passeriformes*). Among the former, we pay special attention to some genera belonging to the family *Fringillidae*, and in addition, to Old World Sparrows (family *Passeridae*, subfamily *Passerinae*, genus *Passer*). Figures 3, 6 and 8 are overviews of the evolutive radiations studied in this chapter.

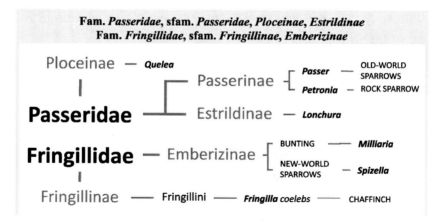

Figure 3. Overview of *Passerinae* evolutive radiations studied in this chapter.

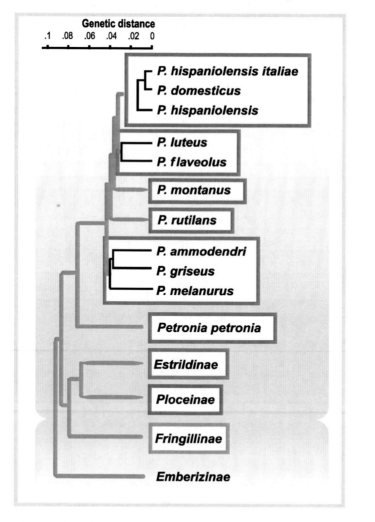

Figure 4. *Passer* species in a linearized tree in relation to other *Passeridae* evolutive groups [13].

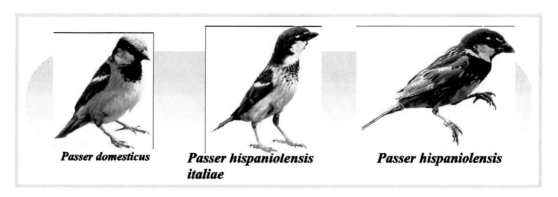

Passer domesticus   *Passer hispaniolensis italiae*   *Passer hispaniolensis*

Figure 5. The P. hispaniolensis italiae case.

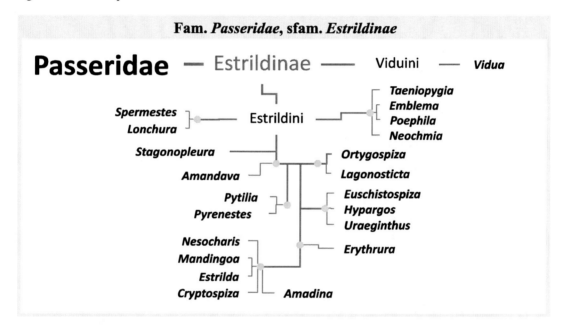

Figure 6. Overview of *Estrildinae* radiations studied in this chapter, according to a Bayesian phylogenetic tree [22].

Many of these species are familiar to man and some of them (canaries) have become a very popular world-wide pet because of the beautiful established color mutations and their strong and beautiful singing. In addition, the red canary (Figure 1) was the first animal obtained by genetic engineering in 1930 in Bremen (Germany) by the conjoint work of a small bird breeder and a geneticist [4].

Some species of Old World sparrows are human commensals in Eurasia and have also been introduced in America and Oceania by European colonists. On the other hand, the establishing of a time of appearance on Earth of birds has been based on a molecular clock calibration which includes both molecular and fossil record data of chicken and pheasant; this was considered the most correct methodology by Vincek et al [5]. Chicken and pheasant separated in Middle Miocene (about 19 MYA [6]) and their Cyt-b DNA sequences were obtained by Zoorob et al. [7]. It was calculated by a mixed molecular/geological clock. This hypothetical time of divergence was used to root most of the trees and divergence between Passerine lines obtained was also validated by Krajewski and King [8], and Fehrer [9].

Once 19 MYA was established as pheasant/chicken divergence time [10], chaffinch (*Fringilla coelebs*) was sometimes used as a precursor and outgroup of other *Fringillidae* because chaffinch is considered more primitive ancestral to other *Fringillinae* birds (it has no crop [11]). It appeared on Earth about 17.5 MYA [10].

In the present chapter, we review (and advance) most of our and other's original work of small songbird familiar to many people, i.e.: sparrows, canaries, goldfinches, and allied. We have tried to draw some conclusions based on genetic phylograms and biogeography to the world of songbirds which have been largely overlooked in this respect. Thus, this chapter may not only be useful for animal geneticists, but also for all small bird breeders. This is because we have avoided much technical language (particularly methodological) that can be found in references and appendix for scholars who need them.

Initial non DNA sequence based classifications have mainly been taken from [3,12], and also changes have been pointed out, according to ours and others' results.

Finally, the birds which are going to be studied in the present chapter have both a great scientific and social impact for humans.

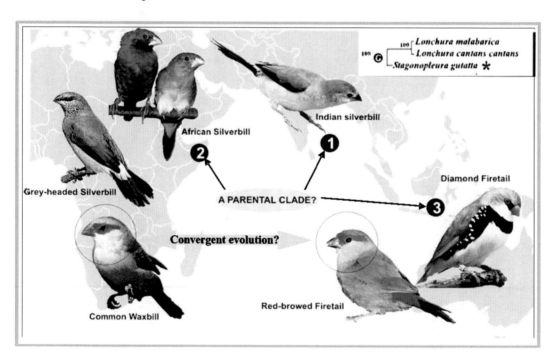

Figure 7. Evolution. Estrildids distribution range. Africa, South Asia (including Arabian Peninsula) and Indonesia, Australia and Pacific Islands. A possible original clade in India is represented. African Silverbill (*Lonchura cantans cantans*) and Indian Silverbill (*Lonchura malabarica*) also thrive in the tip of Arabian Peninsula. African waxbills (genus *Estrilda*) do not have genetic connection with Australian Red-browed Firetail (*Neochmia temporalis*). Grey-headed Silverbill (*Spermestes caniceps* or *Lonchura griseicapilla*) does not cluster with other silverbills (*L. malabarica*, *L. cantans*). Inset shows what may represent Estrildids' parental clade, since it seems the oldest one and is distributed through Africa, India and Australia [22].

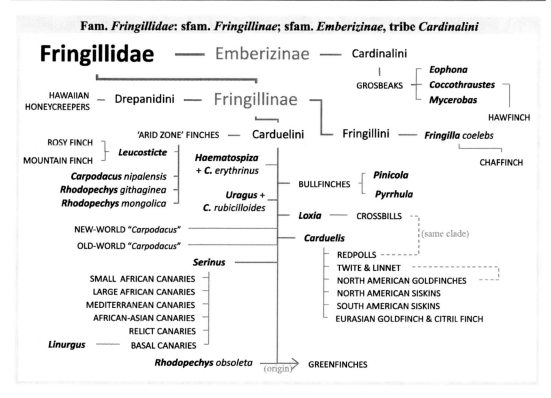

Figure 8. Overview of the *Fringillidae* radiations studied in this chapter. *Fringilla coelebs* is frequently used as outgroup when performing phylogenetic analyses.

PARALLEL *FRINGILLIDAE* AND *PASSERIDAE* EVOLUTIVE RADIATIONS

A continuum of small songbird parallel speciation events among suborder *Passeri* [3,12] are found during Miocene and Pliocene Epochs. Next, we closely examine the evolutive history of *Estrildinae* and *Fringillinae* finches, as well as Old World sparrows (genus *Passer*).

A. Old World Sparrows (fam. *Passeridae*, sfam. *Passerinae*, gen. *Passer*)

The complete geographical range of Old World sparrows distribution has been covered in our studies in African and Eurasian species [13]. House sparrow (*Passer domesticus*) has been introduced throughout the World by man [11,14].

1. Main conclusions about the genetic relatedness among old world sparrows and others

The conclusions about the much debated genetic relationships within Old World sparrows [11,14] are the following:

- The origin of genus *Passer* seems to be African, because the highest number of extant species is African and our phylogenetic results are also suggestive of an African origin; this is in accordance with Summers-Smith [14]. *P. melanurus* or other related extinct species might be the parental one (Figure 4).
- *P. melanurus* (Cape sp arrow) is found to be related to the grey-headed African sparrows and also to *P. ammodendri* (Saxaul sparrow). All three species males have grey melanin pigmentation in the head crown and nape at different degrees. Also, *P. domesticus* may be included in the grey-headed sparrows because of its grey head crown, although no precise placement is found in our phylogenetic trees, probably because more grey-headed African species need to be studied.
- *P. hispaniolensis italiae* (brown-headed sparrow) is probably a *P. domesticus* (grey-head crown) subspecies according to our Unweighted Pair Group With Arithmetic Mean (UPGMA, Figure 4), Neighbor Joining (NJ), and Maximum Parsimony (MP) dendrograms [13] and not a *P. hispaniolensis* subspecies (brown head). This is in accordance with the classical view, but not with more recent opinions [14]. *P. h. italiae* (brown head) may have arisen from *P. domesticus* (grey head crown) by hybridization with *P. hispaniolensis* or any form of divergent speciation [13].

Origin and Other Comments about Genus *Passer*

Timing of the radiation is hypothesized to have run in parallel with other *Passeridae* (rock sparrow, weaverbirds), *Emberizinae* (New and Old World, Figure 4), and *Fringillinae* subfamilies (*Fringillini*, *Carduelini*, (Figure 9). *Passer* radiation could have started in Miocene Epoch. The genus is likely to have appeared in Africa because of the highest number of extant species on this continent [14]. *P. melanurus* is the oldest extant species [13]: it would have been the origin of grey-headed African sparrow species (including *P. domesticus*) and also yellow and other Palearctic bab-sparrows. It has been postulated that the bab-sparrows have probably arisen at the Nile or Rift Valley and followed the human expansion towards Eurasia, giving rise to all Eurasian bab species [14]. This happening would be more feasible if the human expansion had occurred much earlier than thought (5 million years ago), and these birds would have followed it. *P. rutilans* (Asia) seems to be the oldest of the Eurasian sparrows, although its phylogenetic placing within the genus is not clearly defined [13]. The genus *Passer* is strongly associated with man, since most of species nest on man-made buildings and are man commensals [14].

The African grey-headed (*P. grisseus*) and black-headed (*P. melanurus*) sparrows together with the Saxaul sparrow (*P. ammodendri*) seem to form a different clade in relation to the other sparrows. This clade seems the earliest to have originated. No clear geological event is recorded by this time, which may be about 14 MYA in Miocene Epoch [13].

The five species of African grey sparrows may all belong to one species [14]. The only grey species studied by us (*P. grisseus*) is related to the Cape Sparrow (*P. melanurus*), the latter living only in the southern Sahara African range where grey sparrows do not thrive (except *P. diffusus*).

P. melanurus

South African *P. melanurus* (Cape sparrow) clusters together with the African species *P. grisseus* (grey-headed sparrow). *P. luteus* lives in Africa in a land band just below the Sahara

Desert (Sahel) from the East to the West Coast [14]); its position in the phylogenetic trees is ambiguous.

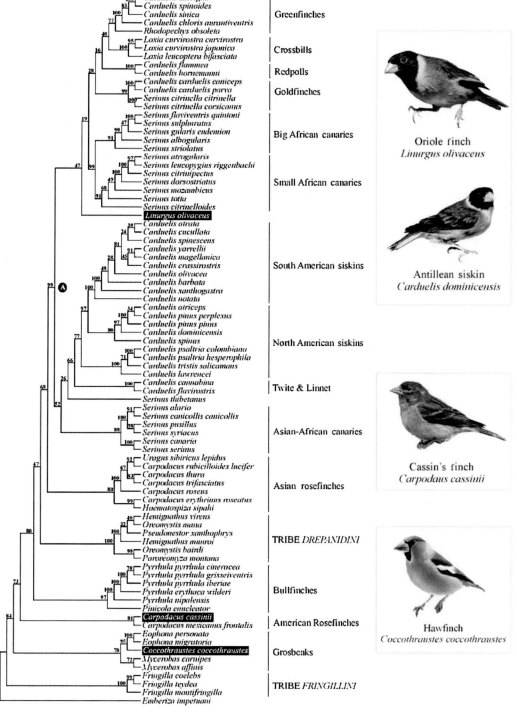

Figure 9a. Linearized Bayesian phylogeny tree based on mitochondrial cytochrome b DNA sequences [25].

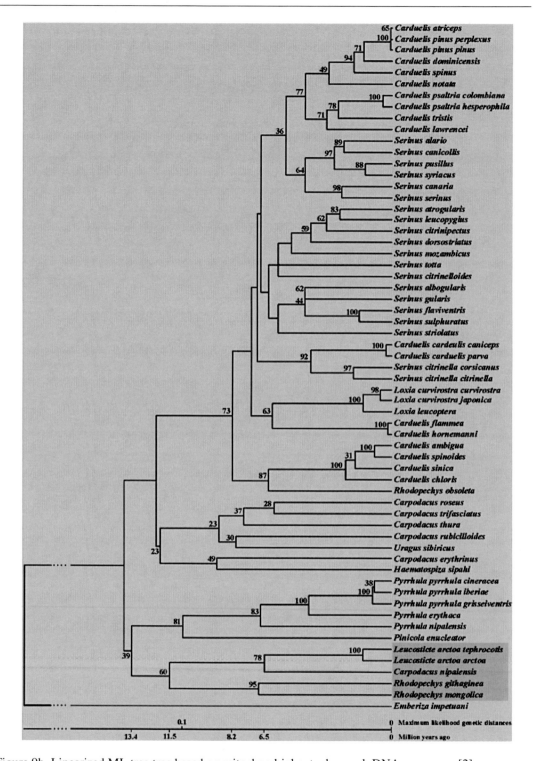

Figure 9b. Linearized ML tree tree based on mitochondrial cytochrome b DNA sequences [2].

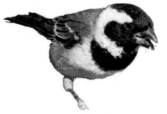
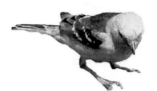

Passer melanurus   **Passer luteus**

It may or may not be closely related to the other African sparrows. However, it is clear that the claims that *P. luteus* does not belong to genus *Passer* is not supported by our genetic data. It may have originated in Sudan and might have expanded from West to East following the hunter-gathered Cushitic people emigration [14,15] as a commensal. *P. ammodendri* (the single sparrow species, other than *P. melanurus*, that has a black nape) is tightly linked to *P. melanurus*; this could have given rise to mutation(s) that diluted melanin at various parts of the head and body and could have originated the grey-headed sparrows, including the *P. grisseus* group—*P. ammodendri* and *P. domesticus* (grey-patched head). *P. ammodendri* is now restricted to the Asian deserts but may have also been originated in Africa and inhabited its deserts in the past, like *P. simplex* (with which it shares a common living range in Asia) [14]. *P. ammodendri* may have been displaced by a recent introduction of *P. simplex* in Africa. Passer domesticus is also a grey-hooded sparrow.

The P. hispaniolensis italiae Classification

Passer domesticus and *P. hispaniolensis* cannot be distinguished osteologically and their ancestor may have appeared 4 MYA. Fossil evidence for this precursor is found 350,000 years ago in Palestine [14]. However, the Pleistocene origin for sparrows and other Passerines (including *Serinus* and *Carduelis* [10,16,17]) could be placed much further back into the Miocene or Pliocene Epochs, Pleistocene being more important in subspeciation. Figure 4 suggests that *P. domesticus* and *P. hispaniolensis* subspeciation may have occurred in the Pleistocene. However, passerine appearance times are still much debated and a Pleistocene origin for species is also suggested [18,19]. Our results report that *P. h. italiae* is a *P. domesticus* subspecies [13].

2. Relationships of Old World Sparrows with Other Genera

The relationships of Old World sparrows radiation to other *Passeridae*: Old and New World *Emberizinae* sparrows, weaver birds (*Ploceinae*), and *Estrildinae* have been studied. Parallel radiations are observed. Rock sparrow (genus *Petronia*) is the closest relative studied to Old World sparrows within the Subfamily *Passerinae*. African *Passeridae*, *Lonchura cucullata* (*Estrildinae*), and *Quelea cardinalis* (a weaver-bird, *Ploceinae*) do not cluster together in dendrograms [13]. Genus *Passer* is not included within the *Ploceinae* in contrast to the suggestion of previous studies in which they were included within weavers (*Ploceinae*) by some authors based mainly on skeletal characters, nest building, and DNA hybridization [14]. *Emberizinae* are also separate from *Passer* in spite of suggestions to join both families according to egg-white protein studies [14]. *Fringilla coelebs* (the cropless chaffinch) is closer to *Lonchura* and *Quelea* than to the *Emberizinae*. It is clear from the phylogenetic trees that Old and New World *Emberizinae* sparrows represent a separate (and single) radiation compared to both *Passeridae* family and Chaffinches (*Fringillidae*) [13].

B. *Estrildinae* Finches (fam. *Passeridae*, sfam. *Estrildinae*)

Both tribes of *Estrildinae* finches (*Estrildini* and *Viduini*) are clearly separated suggesting the monophyly of each group [13,20], contrary to others' suggestion [21]. However, the *Estrildinae* group is composed itself of different evolutive radiations (Figure 6). *Estrildinae* birds thrive in a wide arch comprising Africa, Continental South Asia, Australia and some Indic and Pacific Ocean Islands (Figure 7).

1. Tempo of evolution and origin in the indian subcontinent
Once it is established the monophyly of the *Estrildini* clade ([22], Arnaiz-Villena et al., unpublished), it is feasible to address an approximation of the time of appearance of extant estrildids. A ML linearized tree was calibrated for times by taking into account a mixed chicken/pheasant molecular and geological divergence and then a further calculation for *Fringilla coelebs* and *Sylvia atricapilla* [10]. The estrildid radiation would have started about 16.5 MYA.

The Indian plate crashed against the Asian plate 50 MYA, but the 'strongest push' occurred during the Miocene Epoch [23,24]. As a consequence, the Himalayan peaks established, the Tibetan plateau reached nearly its nowadays altitude and climate changes happened in the Indian peninsula and Himalayan mountains (monsoon rains), and in the Tibetan plateau (colder and drier). The biggest rivers in India, Indochina and China established (starting at Tibetan Plateau) and this climate change may have pushed the *Estrildinae* birds' ancestor to radiate and give rise to present day species (Figures 6, 7) [24]. This fact would suggest an Indian origin for the extant Estrildids, which would have colonized Africa, Australia, South Asia and the Indian and South Pacific Islands, because branch leading to the evolutive group —*Lonchura cantans cantans* (Africa), *Lonchura malabarica* (India), *Stagonopleura guttata* (Australia) — is the oldest one found, basal to others and possible origin of other *Estrildinae* radiations (see Figure 6 and [22]).

2. Specific phylogenetic problems addressed

Genera Estrilda and Nesocharis
The Grey-headed oliveback (*Nesocharis capistrata*), and presumably the two other *Nesocharis* species, *N. shelleyi* and *N. ansorgei* (not tested), groups with *Estrilda* species in a basal branch (except *E. melanotis*), and seems to be older than the *Estrilda* species (Figure 6). Although more taxa are required, it is likely that genus *Estrilda* and genus *Nesocharis* belong to the same radiation and could be considered as members of the same genus, despite the remarkably different phenotype.

Gouldian Finch

The popular pet Gouldian Finch (*Chloebia gouldiae* / *Erythrura gouldiae*) is definitively included within the bright colored birds of genus *Erythrura*, according to our Bayesian analyses.

Silverbills

Silverbills from genus *Lonchura* have been suggested to cluster together and separated from other *Lonchura* species [11]. This fact is partially confirmed by our results, showing the oldest Estrildinae evolutive radiation group that consistently clusters the African silverbill (*Lonchura cantans*) with the Indian silverbill (*Lonchura malabarica*), and also with the phenetically distinct Diamond Firetail (*Stagonopleura guttata*) from Australia. This group is not related to the rest of 'non-silverbill' *Lonchura* species. Another silverbill, however (the Grey-headed Silverbill, *Spermestes caniceps*), is placed within a different cluster, the *Spermestes* one.

Java Sparrow (*Padda oryzivora* / *Lonchura oryzivora*)

The Java sparrow might be considered a *Lonchura* species according to our Bayesian and Maximum Likelihood (ML) analyses.

•African Munias

The African munias show a distinct phylogenetic cluster with respect to the Asian and Australian munias, corroborating the distinction proposed by some authors [3], who designate the former as belonging to the genus *Spermestes* and keep the latter as members of the genus *Lonchura* [3,12].

Plum-headed Finch (*Aidemosyne modesta* / *Neochmia modesta*)

The Plum-headed Finch clusters in our analyses with other Australian finches, close to *Neochmia* and *Poephila* species, as previously seen [20,21].

Red-browed Firetail (*Aegintha* / *Neochmia temporalis*)

Clement, in the Introduction of his 1993 edition [11], pointed out that the Australian Red-browed Firetail was very similar to some African waxbills from genus *Estrilda* (Figure 6). We have seen that it appears as a basal species of all *Estrildinae* birds in our Bayesian analysis, but it is integrated among the Australian group in the ML tree, i.e. *Poephila* spp., *Taeniopygia guttata*, *Neochmia ruficauda clarescens*, *Neochmia modesta*, *Emblema pictum*, *Taeniopygia bichenovii*) [22]. In any case, it is not genetically related to the African waxbills, and the red eye brow may be due to convergent evolution driven by unknown evolutive forces. The Australian red-browed firetail is probably an ancestral Australian estrildid (Figure 7).

Cryptospiza Radiation

A group that clusters together *Mandingoa nitidula*, *Cryptospiza reichenovii* and *Estrilda melanotis* with a low statistical support is found. However, we think that *Mandingoa nitidula* and *Estrilda melanotis* may be joined to genus *Cryptospiza*.

Other Estrildid species, like *Pyrenestes sanguineus*, *Lagonostica senegala*, *Ortygospiza atricollis*, *Hypargos niveoguttatus*, *Euschistospiza dybowskii* and *Emblema pictum* show a similar (but not clearly resolved) grouping, as previously suggested [20,21].

Regarding the geographical distribution range, we do not find a genetic separation between the African and Australian Estrildids, being all of them intermixed in various phylogenetic groups [22]. Figure 7 shows present day estrildid range. Three questions are addressed in this figure:

(1) A hypothetical original place of estrildids may be India.
(2) Silverbills do not cluster together.
(3) Wallace's Line is drawn between the Indonesian Islands of Bali and Lombok (both of them known as part of the Lesser Sunda Islands), and also between Borneo and Sulawesi (former Celebes) Islands to mark the boundary between the Oriental and Australian regions. The Wallace's line corresponds almost exactly with the outer limit of the continental shelf of South Asia. This was exposed by lowered sea level during Pleistocene glaciations [24]. Although many species of birds, mammals and plants are mostly thriving either at one or the other side of the line because of the relative dispersal barrier before Asian shelf during Pleistocene glaciations, no particular speciation of dispersal event is noticed around Pleistocene, 2 MYA and after (Figure 6). This indicates that Estrildids speciation and radiation had occurred before Pleistocene, starting after 16.5 MYA (Figure 6).

C. Carduelini Finches (fam. *Fringillidae*, sfam. *Fringillinae*, tribe *Carduelini*)

Both tribes *Drepanidini* and *Fringillini* (Figure 8) form distinct well-defined monophyletic groups, according to the Bayesian analysis (Figure 9a), while tribe *Carduelini* seems to comprise a number of paraphyletic groups (Figure 10, which is a scheme of Figure 9a) [21,25].

The estimated divergence time for most of genus *Carduelis* species suggests that they appeared in a range of time between the Miocene and Pliocene; there is no evidence for a divergence time consistent with late Pleistocene origin for most radiation groups [22]. This radiation was intermingled in time with *Serinus* species radiation (Bayesian dendrogram in Figure 9a, ML tree in Figure 9b) [2,25].

However, it is possible that certain *Carduelis* birds, classically considered as subspecies, originated during Pleistocene glaciations; the divergence time calculated for *C. carduelis* subspecies (grey-headed Asian and black-headed European goldfinch) is less than 800,000 years [2,10]. Also, late glaciations may have separated western European siskins (*C. spinus*) from the Far East subspecies by an ice-induced vicariance event. In conclusion, the lack of evidence found by others [26] for Pleistocene speciation in North American songbirds has also been found in the present study not only in North America but also in Eurasia and South American siskins. Indeed, the analysis of most extant species of genus *Serinus* supports the same conclusions about time of radiations and subspecies, and includes the African southern Hemisphere for *Serinus* [17].

Crossbills, bullfinches, grosbeaks, and "*Carpodacus*" studied species may have arisen between the Miocene and Pliocene Epochs [2,10,25]. However, although these appearance times have been found for *Serinus* and *Carduelis* [2,10,17], these early timings for passerine emergence are accepted by most [5,16,27] but not by all [19] authors.

1. Genus Carduelis

Only 4% average amount of nucleotide substitution per lineage is found between the most distantly related of the 25 *Carduelis* species [10]. This suggests a relatively fast radiation of this genus, compared to other documented songbird radiations (i.e. genus *Zonotrichia*, 4.1% for only 7 species; genus *Pipilo*, 6.4% for only 6 species [28,29]).

A tentative classification might be proposed for genus *Carduelis* that takes into account our molecular phylogenetic data [10,30] and also geographical and gross phenotypic data, that is, body size. We suggest the following group classification:

- Eurasian Goldfinch (*Carduelis carduelis*) and Citril Finch (*Carduelis citrinella*, formerly *Serinus citrinella* [12])
- Greenfinches
- Twite (*Carduelis flavirostris*) and Linnet (*Carduelis cannabina*). Genus *Acanthis* including twite, linnet and redpolls could be abandoned as a taxonomic unit; twite and linnet are in some dendrograms significantly close to North American *Carduelis tristis* radiation.
- North American Goldfinch (*Carduelis tristis*)
- North American Siskins
- South American Siskins (from North American ancestor *C. notata*)
- Northern Redpolls (*Carduelis flammea* and *Carduelis hornemanni*) and Crossbills

Eurasian Goldfinch (*Carduelis carduelis*) and Citril Finch (*Carduelis citrinella*)

Phylogeny dendrograms of most *Carduelis* [10] and *Serinus* [17] genera extant species show that both radiations are intermingled in time and that both genera are polyphyletic [31]; the earliest *Serinus* species seem to have appeared in the Miocene Epoch about 9 MYA, slightly after the first *Carduelis* species (about 9.5 MYA) [31], possibly in the Asian continent and coinciding with dramatic changes of the climate when the eastern Mediterranean (*Tethis*) Sea was closing [32-34]. Pleistocene glaciations may have induced further speciation events but on a scale lower than previously thought (Figure 10) [16].

Classical goldfinches (Figure 11) comprise the European black-headed goldfinch (*C. carduelis*, with some subspecies, like South European *C. c. parva*) and the Asian (grey-headed) goldfinch (*C. c. caniceps, major*, and others) [11]. Both grey- and black-headed subspecies include variants with a marked degree of local differences in size, beak, shape and colors. *Serinus citrinella* (citril finch, classified before as a canary) is a relict of a few Mediterranean islands (Corsica, Sardinia) and central and southern European mountains; it has been found to be a close relative to goldfinches and may be classified as such, since both have common ancestors. This bird has been renamed *Carduelis citrinella* [12] The ancestor of these species may have appeared around 6 MYA. Color, body and bill shape of citril finch are very different from these of typical goldfinches; however, its singing, which is delivered in short repeated phrases with metallic notes, is similar to that of classical goldfinches (*Carduelis carduelis*) and the type of flight (light and undulating) resembles that of the goldfinch (our own observations; [11]). Color and shape of beak have been shown to evolve very rapidly in birds, even in a range of hundreds of years [35].

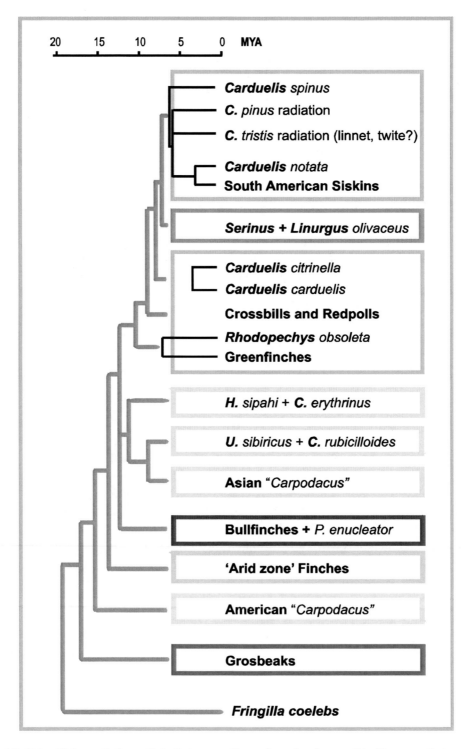

Figure 10. *Fringillidae* radiations. Note that genus *Carpodacus* has been split off on genetic bases [2,10,17,25,44].

a. European Citril Finch: Islands and Continent

   Citril finch island individuals seem to be more ancient than those extant in the continent.

   The taxonomic status of citril finch (*Carduelis citrinella*) as a canary has been questioned on molecular, behavioral and phenotypic bases [10,17,36]. However, Francisco Bernis [37] named it *Carduelis citrinella* based on phenotypic, behavioral and biogeographic characters [12]. Today, it is generally accepted as the Eurasian goldfinch ancestor [12,31].

   A controversy has also arisen about assigning separate species status to the insular "Koenig" type, *S. c. corsicanus* (Corsica, Sardinia, and Tuscany islands) and to the mainland or "Pallas" type, *S. c. citrinella* (Pyrenees, Alps, and Spanish northern and Central mountains [38]). Both forms show phenotypic differences [11,31,39] and, particularly, the brown back is typical of the island species against the grey mantle of the continental ones. Also, singing is different between the two citril finch forms [39-41]. Pasquet and Thibault [41] suggested that the divergence of continental and island forms may be more recent than the last connection between the mainland and the Sardinia-Corsica complex during the Messinian salinity crisis. On the other hand, they did not find significant genetic divergence of mtDNA to consider mainland and insular forms as two different species [31]. However, Sangster [42] pointed out that intra- and interspecies percentage of genetic citril finch divergence overlap; our results [30,31] suggest that *C. citrinella* from the islands gave rise to continental form.

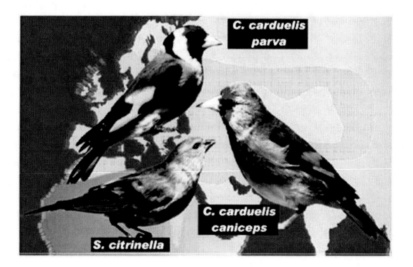

Figure 11. Eurasian goldfinches [10;41].

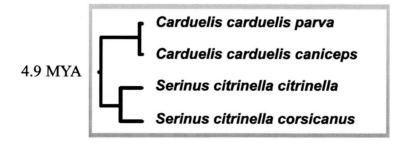

Figure 12. The particular case of *Carduelis citrinella* (ML tree) [12,17,41,42].

Citril finch seems to have diverged from European goldfinches about 5 MYA, and later (2.6 MYA) the divergence between mainland and insular *C. citrinella* forms may have occurred (Figure 12). All phylogenetic analyses show that the insular forms (subspecies) of *C. citrinella* share the most recent ancestor with *C. carduelis*, in contrast to the continental forms. We do not find behavioral, phonetic, or genetic data enough to change *C. citrinella corsicana* from subspecies to species status, separate from *C. citrinella citrinella* [31].

The island citril finch forms are genetically closer to the hypothesized goldfinch / citril finch common ancestor, this is confirmed by both distance and cladistic methodologies [30,31]; however, more citril finch individuals need to be studied. It is possible that some intermediate species between these two sister groups are now extinct. If *Carduelis* and *Serinus* radiations took place in the Miocene Epoch (Figure 10) [10,17], the divergence of both citril finch forms could have been coincidental with the Messinian salinity crisis [41]. Thus, an evolutionary hypothesis could be that an ancestor evolved to a form of citril finch (*C. corsicanus*) in Corsica or Sardinia about 5 MYA when the Gibraltar Strait closed, the Mediterranean Sea dried up and an arid climate established. Only salty mountains and very salty small lakes there existed in the western Mediterranean basin [43]. The Mediterranean Sea filled with water again about half million years later. It may be postulated that an ancestral finch (to the citril finch forms) got isolated in the Sardinian or Corsican mountains during the arid period [43] having the only available source of non-salty drinking water there. This island citril finch could have resulted from a vicariate speciation there, keeping brown back, like its sister species (the European goldfinch), and probably like a common ancestor(s) [31,44]. Later, *S. c. corsicanus* could have reached the continental mountains, Alps and others, through the "Toscana islands" and would have later lost the brown back, becoming the *S. c. citrinella* form. This may have also reached the Iberian mountains. Other hypotheses are not discarded.

Grey- and dark-headed goldfinch subspecies have probably split during Pleistocene glaciations less than 1 MYA, when eastern (grey-headed) and western (black-headed) goldfinch ancestors may have become isolated probably by ice-caused vicariance events. In general, Pleistocene glaciations are shown not to be related to *Carduelis* or *Serinus* [10,17,31] speciation around the world (including the Southern Hemisphere): pre-Pleistocene glaciations speciation of songbirds is also found by Klicka and Zink for North America (northern hemisphere) by studying other *Passerine* genera [26].

b. Greenfinches (C. chloris, C. sinica, C. ambigua and C. spinoides)

They seem to be the earliest appeared lineage belonging to the genus *Carduelis*; their ancestors probably originated around 9 MYA [44], together with *Rhodopechys obsoleta*, an identified extant ancestor of greenfinches [44], at the time when Mediterranean Sea started drying up and the climate around the sea also got drier. Only *C. chloris* (greenfinch) lives in Europe and North Africa. Greenfinches are the *Carduelis* finches closest to the outgroup *Fringilla coelebs* (chaffinch), and *C. ambigua* and *C. spinoides* may have originated from the same ancestor by ice-caused vicariance during the last 2 MY glaciations, although their ancestors could have existed 9 MYA [44].

c. Desert Finch

Greenfinches: Desert Finch (*Rhodopechys obsoleta*) as ancestor of Eurasian Greenfinches (*C. chloris, C. sinica, C. ambigua, C. spinoides*)

Biogeographic (Global Warming) Hypothesis

While *R. githaginea* and *R. mongolica* would have arisen about 6.8 MYA (Figure 32), *R. obsoleta* (desert finch) appeared about 8 MYA, and seems to be a closely related ancestor of the greenfinches lineage, which started about 9 MYA (figs, 10, 13) in the Miocene Epoch. Indeed, about 7–5 MYA, a glacial mantle covered Antarctica and Greenland and many Asian and African arid areas appeared [23]. About 2.6 MYA, when the weather became much warmer [23] and during periods of severe drought, bordering populations of desert finch might have set out from semi-desert areas to more humid habitats and evolved to a greenfinch-like bird (extant or extinct ancestor). This ancestor may have differently evolved in Western Europe and Eastern Asia giving rise to *C. chloris* and *C. sinica*, respectively (Figure 13). Later, during the climate changes of the last 2 MYA glaciations [23], *C. sinica* populations may have dispersed southwards giving rise to *C. ambigua* and, finally, populations of this latter species would have also dispersed evolving to *C. spinoides* [10].

Whether *R. obsoleta* also existed in African deserts remains as a possibility. Also, an African *R. obsoleta* ancestor for the Mediterranean-European greenfinch (*C. chloris*) is not discarded.

Evolutionary Pattern Hypothesis

The question arises as to how the speciation leading to greenfinches from a semi-desert-based species like *R. obsoleta* or a close extinct species would have proceeded. The answer could be related to the different environments in which greenfinches and desert finch might have occurred. Open habitats (i.e., deserts or arid-areas) inhabited by *Rhodopechys* spp., are thought to favor pale color and lower bright values in plumage colorations than do other habitats [45]. Sandy and pale colored wings could be mirroring a convergent evolution to a desert environment adaptation between *R. mongolica* / *R. githaginea* and *R. obsoleta* (Figure 14). Conversely, *R. obsoleta*'s molecular sister taxa (greenfinches) bear olive green, bright green and bright yellow plumages that usually result from melanin and carotenoid pigment combinations [35].

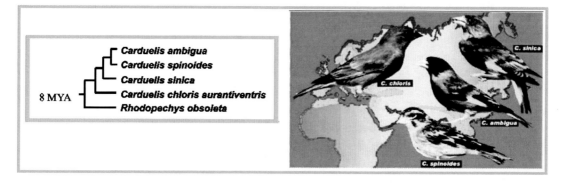

Figure 13. Greenfinches [10,44].

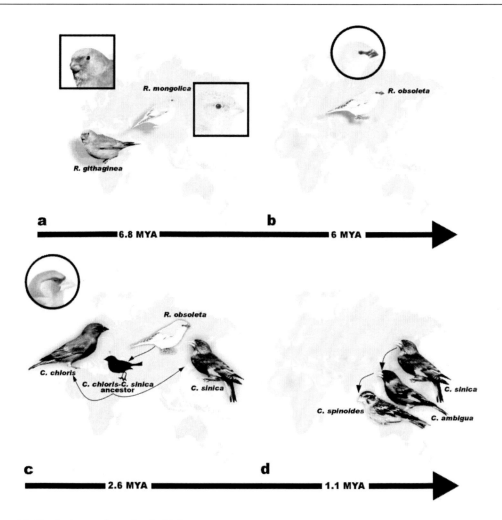

Figure 14. Evolutionary hypothesis [44].

C. atriceps in orange; *C. p. perplexus* in purple. Inset represents a Bayesian Inference dendrogram based on mitochondrial cytochrome b DNA sequences. Note that the nodes are strongly supported independently of the methodology used.

These colorations may provide a better species-specific signaling performance in denser habitats, such as forests or other non-arid areas. Melanin pigments have been considered to protect feathers from bacterial degradation in humid habitats [46]. Thus, higher melanin content may have been selected in populations settling down in forests or similar more humid habitats (i.e., in greenfinches).

Other melanin related characters, like the eye-stripe present in both *R. obsoleta* and *C. Chloris* males, may contribute to sexual dimorphism and female mating choice in the breeding season (see head details in Figure 13). This would suggest that the extant closest relative to *R. obsoleta* is *C. chloris*, which is the only one with a preserved black eye-stripe in the breeding season. Carotenoids, the other major pigments responsible for plumage colorations [35], are scarce in dry areas, and could have reduced to a minimum in the diet of species occurring in Central Asia or Africa areas undergoing desertification in Pliocene and

Miocene Epochs. In this way, adaptive convergence to a sandy and pale color plumage common in the traditionally recognized *Rhodopechys* species could have occurred in *R. obsoleta* via carotenoid shortage, among other environmental factors [46].

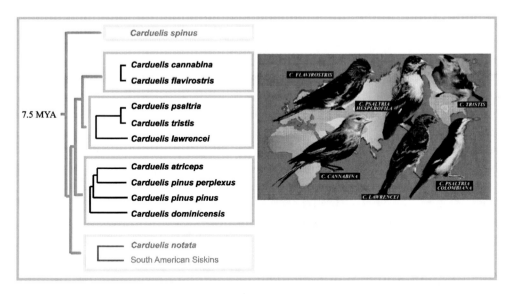

Figure 15. North American siskin radiation; linnet and twite [10,30].

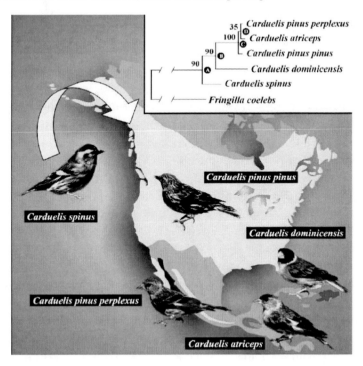

Figure 16. The Eurasian Siskin (*Carduelis spinus*) possibly thrived in North America before two million years ago when glaciations started. The ice shield on North America could have driven speciation by provincialism of 'daughter species' isolated in the Caribbean Mountains (*C. dominicensis*), in Mexican Sierras (*C. p. pinus*) and in Mexican-Guatemalan altiplano (*C. p. perplexus* and *C. atriceps*) [30]. Present day ranges: *C. p. pinus* in yellow; *C. dominicensis* in red.

On the other hand, the assortative mating selection may not only be restricted to differences in feather pigment content; species specific song may also influence the assortative mating [47,48] between allopatric populations of *R. obsoleta* which may later have differentiated into species (*R. obsoleta* and *C. chloris*). *R. obsoleta* song, although more harsh and nasal, is similar to those of *C. chloris* and the linnet (*Carduelis cannabina*, Europe and western Asia) [49].

Twite (Carduelis flavirostris) and Linnet (Carduelis cannabina): Related to American Goldfinches?

Both parsimony and NJ dendrograms (Figure 15) separate several groups which are in general concordant with present-day geographical distributions [10] ; however, there are some important exceptions. Siskin (*C. spinus*, Eurasia) and pine siskin (*C. pinus*, North America) are grouped together (Figures 15, 16). These sister species may also be related to another group which comprises a surprising mixture of North American and Eurasian species. The Eurasian ones are *C. cannabina* (linnet) and its sister species *C. flavirostris* (twite), which do not appear to form a group (so-called *Acanthis*) with *C. flammea* (common redpoll) and *C. hornemanni* (Arctic redpoll), as had been proposed [50]. Also, the lineage leading to both redpolls, which inhabit northern areas, may have appeared approximately 9 MYA, while that leading to twite and linnet may have arisen about 2 MY later. The attachment of linnet and twite to North American goldfinches (c. tristis evolutive radiation) does not occur in all dendrograms [10,31], and might represent a single radiation (Figure 10, 15) with disappeared ancestors.

North American *Carduelis* Radiations

Eurasian siskin (*C. spinus*) could have been the ancestor of all American *Carduelis* species, because it is the only one Eurasian *Carduelis* that has a clear and distinct genetic relationship with one of the three extant American *Carduelis* radiations: the **pine siskin** radiation [30,51]. The other two American finch radiations, i.e.: **C. tristis** and **C. notata** ones have lost a genetic link with *C. spinus* if they ever had one.

However, a particular Major Histocompatibility Complex protein allele (Arnaiz-Villena A, unpublished), which was present in a *C. spinus* (5 MYA) individual [10,31] from the Pyrenees Mountains (North Spain), was also present in *C. atrata* (0.5 MYA), an endemic South American siskin living at 5000 meters of altitude around Andean Titicaca Lake and close-by areas.

Nowadays, the Eurasian Siskin does not thrive in America, but in easternmost and westernmost Eurasia, leaving a gap between Central Russia and its easternmost range. The most important feature of the Eurasian Siskin is that it is a migratory bird whose North to South migrations do not always follow the same longitudinal patterns ("irruptive") [11]. It is feasible that *Carduelis spinus* was thriving in Eurasia and also in North America around the Pliocene / Pleistocene Epoch limit, about 2 MYA. Soon after this time, the first Glaciation covered North America with a kilometric thick ice shield [30,51]. The Eurasian Siskin might have taken refuge in ice-free Caribbean Islands and in Mexican Mountains and Guatemalan-Mexican altiplano. Its Summer-Winter and North-South migrations would have been disrupted because it became isolated in all-year relatively warm temperature (Caribbean); year-round relatively and quite stable low temperature (Guatemalan-Mexican altiplano) and relatively stable temperature in Mexican Mountains. The Eurasian Siskin could have first given rise to the endemic Antillean Siskin (*Carduelis dominicensis*) at the Caribbean high peaks of La Hispaniola Island soon after 2 MYA (Figure 16) [30,52]. Afterward, about 200,000 years ago, the Eurasian Siskin might have given rise to the Pine Siskin *Carduelis pinus pinus* in the non-glaciated Mexican Sierras [30,53]; at about the same time (200,000 years ago), the Black-capped Siskin (*Carduelis atriceps*) and the Pine Siskin *Carduelis pinus perplexus* might have appeared in the non-glaciated Guatemalan-Mexican altiplano [24]. Rainfall variations in the Caribbean during the Pleistocene, however, could have also affected the distribution of these birds [54].

This would be a typical example of adaptive radiation caused by a North to South migration barrier (First North American Ice Shield Glaciation) and provincialism that drove evolution to create these new finch species. When the last Wisconsin Glaciation ended and North American ice melted about 12,000 years ago, *Carduelis pinus* would have followed the ancestral North to South migrations and covered all North America, occupying the American niches that the Eurasian Siskin couldn't reach from Asia during the last 2 million years because of the extant thick ice shield; neither could it afterwards because of species competition by ecologic niche with its descent *Carduelis pinus*. This evolutionary theory for the finch group appearance is schematic. More complicated events may have occurred during the Nebraskan, Kansan, Illinoan and Wisconsin North American glaciations, and/or their respective interglacial periods (Aftonian, Yarmouth and Sangamon), and other explanations may also be possible [55].

a. North American Goldfinch (Carduelis tristis) Radiation: Relationship with Twite and Linnet (Figures 10, 15)

The *C. pinus / C. spinus* group is probably phylogenetically related to North American goldfinches (*C. tristis*, *C. lawrencei* and *C. psaltria*) and possibly to the Eurasian linnet (*C. cannabina*) and twite (*C. flavirostris*), but linking species are missing [10,30]. Siskin and pine siskin may have diverged from a species which lived throughout the Northern Hemisphere probably about 3 MYA; the Bering Strait was not a geographical barrier during long periods in the last 2 MY [32]. North American *Carduelis* finches from this radiation should not be named goldfinches, since they have only a distant molecular relationship with European goldfinches; instead they should be included among siskins. *C. tristis* (American goldfinch) and *C. psaltria* (lesser goldfinch) are also close relatives. The first is found in North America, including parts of Mexico, and the second is thriving in western United States and Mexico (*C. ps. hesperophilus*, green back), in Southwest United States and Central America (*C. ps. psaltria*), and northern South America (*C. ps. colombiana*) down to Peru and the Andean Spine [10,11]; the two latter subspecies show a deep dark back, and hybrids among the three subspecies with the corresponding phenotypic variability have been observed [11]. Although the geographical distribution and phenotype of *C. psaltria* suggest that it could have shared a recent common ancestor with the South American siskins, our results indicate that *C. psaltria* is a North American bird which has colonized South American habitats and has undergone the corresponding phenotypic changes (darker in head and back). An ancestor of *C. psaltria* and *C. tristis* may have existed around 5 MYA; *C. psaltria* subspecies may have originated relatively recently, about 1 MYA. This subspeciation may have occurred after the closing of the Panama Isthmus (5–3 MYA) [10].

b. North American Pine Siskin (Carduelis pinus) Radiation: an Eurasian Ancestor Siskin, Carduelis spinus

We have stated above that taking into account geographic and evolutive parameters, *C. spinus* is the extant common ancestor to all American *Carduelis* birds. Some authors suggest that siskins originated in North America and may have later dispersed to Asia, Europe and South America. Also, the oldest and precursor siskin has been proposed to be *C. pinus*. However, the fact that *C. spinus* is not thriving in North America points to this species being the oldest one. The earliest siskin species are both *C. pinus* and *C. spinus* ancestors together with *C. lawrencei* (6 MYA); *C. tristis* and *C. psaltria* lineages would be slightly more recent (about 5 MYA). However, if the Eurasian twite and linnet are considered akin to North American siskins, they or their ancestors would be the oldest (6.5 MYA) and precursor siskins. It is uncertain but possible that linnet and twite were once living in North America and that Eurasian siskin existed both in America and Eurasia; Bering Strait land bridges have occurred intermittently and may have facilitated exchanges [32].

Siskin, North American Antillean siskin, black-capped siskin, pine siskin and pine siskin perplexus form a monophyletic group separated from other North and South American *Carduelis* spp. (Figure 15). Variability within the Cyt-b gene was sufficient to establish phylogenetic relationships according to the number of observed parsimony-informative sites (146) [56]. Nearly all sequence differences were silent substitutions, as expected [57]: 64.3 % of the third codon positions were not conserved among species, as it has previously been shown for this gene (evolving relatively rapidly under strong functional constraints). The variability for the first and second codon positions was 9.7 % and 2.3 %, respectively, as expected [10,13,17,58].

Eurasian siskin (*C. spinus*) seems to be a close relative to North American *Carduelis* species. This phylogenetic pattern would not fit with its Eurasian distribution range. However, siskin and pine siskin "react" to each other in captivity [39], are closely related [10,59], and are thought to form a superspecies [39,60]. The answers as to why Eurasian siskin does not thrive nowadays in North America and how it gave rise to *C. dominicensis* remain unclear and open to debate, but this has been discussed above. Central to these issues is the fact that West Indies have been continuously colonized primarily by birds from Central America and more recently from South America [35,61-63]. Based on these premises, it is suggested (see also above) that easternmost Asian *Carduelis spinus* passed to America through the Beringia / Aleutian Islands. After this, during the Pliocene Epoch, *C. spinus* invasions from an undetermined area of the North American East coast reached the Antilles and evolved as a geographical isolate resulting in the present *C. dominicensis*. Although phenotypic differences between *C. spinus* and *C. dominicensis* are evident (Figure 16), they may be primarily not entirely based on genetic differences, but also on distinctive environmental forces [64] and/or are controlled by genes with a higher evolutionary rate [65]. The effect of directional selection due to adaptation to new environment and genetic drift may be responsible for the very different phenotype. With regard to the present day absence of *C. spinus* in North America, *C. spinus* has been recorded in the American part of the Bering Strait and in the Aleutian Islands; these have been considered escapes from captivity [11].

Antillean siskin (*Carduelis dominicensis*) was first described by Bryant [66]. The species is monotypic (with no subspecies), endemic to mountain pine forest of Hispaniola Island (Haiti and Dominican Republic [11], which are the highest mountains of the Caribbean Islands.

The time of appearance of Antillean siskin seems to be 2 MYA (Figure 16) [10,30], in the Pliocene Epoch.

A phylogenetic placement of this species within South American siskins was discarded. It seems that Antillean siskin would be the oldest of the North American birds within this group, and that had given rise to pine siskin [30]. Most of the *Carduelis dominicensis* particular traits (black head and neck, yellow breast) [11] are shared with other forest or highland birds like *Carduelis notata* (black-headed siskin) [10,11], *Linurgus olivaceus* (oriole finch) [11,25,30] and *Mycerobas* genus spp. [11]. Thus, these head and color traits in Antillean siskin might be due to convergent evolution on a highland forest.

Pine siskin was first described by Wilson [67]. This species thrives in North America from Alaska, South to Guatemala [11]. mtDNA from pine siskin taken at Dolores (Colorado) was arbitrarily chosen for tree building and calculations (Figure 10) [30], because other single samples from distant sites within the pine siskin range had almost identical sequences. Its origin could be postulated about 200,000 YA, in the late Pleistocene [30]. This species has already been described as a sister taxa of the *Carduelis spinus* [10].

Carduelis pinus perplexus is resident below the Mexican Isthmus in the highlands (2,000-3,500 m) from northern Chiapas to western Guatemala [68]. Our specimens were captured in Quetzaltenango (Guatemala highlands). Pine siskin perplexus is quite different in appearance from pine siskin and studies are necessary to determine its taxonomic status [30,69], although it is genetically closer to *Carduelis atriceps* [30], black-capped siskin.

Black-capped siskin was first described by Salvin [70]. This bird is monotypic (with no different subspecies), from the highlands of Chiapas, southeast Mexico, south to the western highlands of Guatemala. Pine siskin perplexus is grouped with black-capped siskin in the p genetic distance matrix [30] and in analyses that include several individuals of pine siskin and black-capped siskin.

Finally, it appears that siskin, Antillean siskin, pine siskin, pine siskin perplexus and black-capped siskin form a monophyletic group separated from other North American *Carduelis* finches (*C. lawrencei*, *C. tristis*, *C. psaltria*, which seem to be closer to other European *Carduelis* in some trees: twite and linnet [10]. Antillean siskin is not genetically related to South American siskins [10].

It seems that some Museums have original "all-green" *C. atriceps* (Ottaviani M, personal communication). It does not fit with our original capture in Guatemala highlands of an "all-grey" specimen in full breeding rainy station —August— (Figure 16). We believe that the "all-green" birds captured in Guatemala are *Carduelis spinescens nigricauda*, which was vagrant in Guatemala from Colombia and not captured in breeding season (Arnaiz-Villena A, in preparation); or, more likely, the green morph of *Carduelis pinus pinus* vagrant in Guatemala in non-breeding season [11].

c. North / South American Siskin Radiation: a North American Ancestor, Carduelis notata

The extant parental species, C. Notata, thrives in Mexican mountains and itself or some extinct ancestor successfully colonized South America about 3 MYA, giving rise to the South American siskin radiation (Figure 18). They show very close molecular and phenotypic relationships (particularly color distribution and bill shape, Figure 18) and probably originated quite rapidly after the Isthmus of Panama emerged (Figure 17). This is an example of a quick siskin radiation probably due to rapid dispersal into the South American island (isolated between 95 and 5–3 MYA) which had recently joined the North; although small birds can fly long distances [35], it is possible that the South American *Carduelis* radiation occurred only when mesothermal plants (genus *Carduelis* food) from the Rocky Mountains invaded the Andean spine after the emergence of the Isthmus of Panama (Figure 17) [71].

Northern Redpolls (*Carduelis flammea* and *Carduelis hornemanni*): Disappearance of Genus *Acanthis* and Relationship with Crossbills (genus *Loxia*)

Both redpolls, *C. flammea* and *C. hornemanni* (Arctic redpoll), are now considered to be sister subspecies [3,11] and should be separated from twite (*Carduelis flavirostris*) and linnet (*Carduelis cannabina*). They are two different evolutionary radiations, because they:

(i) are the only *Carduelis* species which live all along the Holoarctic region, i.e. North Eurasia and North America (Figure 19)

(ii) do not clearly group together within any other *Carduelis* subgroup (Figure 10), but with genus *Loxia* (crossbills), which may in turn be included within genus *Carduelis* (Figure 19)

(iii) are evolutionarily distant from linnet and twite, which are close to North American siskins (*C. tristis* group) according to parsimony and NJ dendrograms [10]; thus genus *Acanthis*, which included twite, linnet and redpolls, may not exist. It is likely that both redpoll subspecies also separated during Pleistocene glaciations around 500,000 years before present. This date has already been suggested [72]; their ancestors may have lived in the Miocene about 9 MYA [10,58]

Crossbills (genus *Loxia*, Figure 20) are integrated within the genus *Carduelis*, together with redpolls with high bootstrap [10,58]. Common crossbill (*Loxia curvirostra*) shows subspeciation with *L. japonica* in the Pleistocene epoch [58]. Like redpolls, crossbills have a northern hemisphere distribution, and a characteristic crossed mandible for specialized extraction of conifer seeds. They seem to have a more ancient origin than redpolls (Figure 19) [10,58]. They probably originated from a *Carduelis*-like ancestor when conifers were very common on Earth. Pine cones undergo irregular cycles of appearance and redpolls may have evolved at a time when pine cones were scarce and the hypothetical ancestor of the redpoll was forced to emerge from the conifer woods to find food in neighboring small mesothermal plants. The time when this occurred is uncertain; if we take the time scale hypothesized in Figure 19, it would be about 9 MYA. There was clearly a decline in the number of conifers after the cold periods of Pleistocene glaciations, when redpolls could have appeared. However, the time scale is still debated [10,16,17,19,27]. Beak shape may change very rapidly according to feeding needs (i.e., lack of conifers [35]).

The Arctic redpoll (*C. hornemanni*, size 14 cm) has a very similar length to that of *Loxia curvirostra japonica*, a very small *Loxia* subspecies (14–15 cm). Red color varying in distribution placements and intensity according to subspecies, is conserved in both crossbill and redpoll males [11]. Typical seasonal North-South migrating patterns occur in both crossbills and redpolls, but the characteristic southern irruptive behavior of the former is unique, perhaps because the availability of pine cones is unpredictable in the pine woods [11,50].

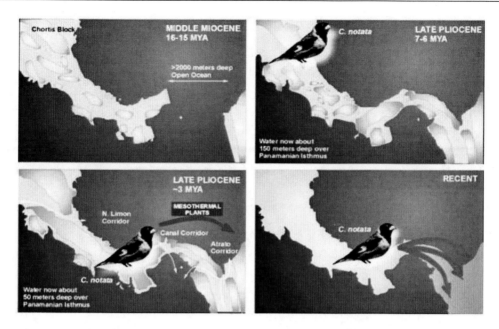

Figure 17. Appearance of South American siskins. Extant *C. notata* or an extinct related species followed mesothermal plants' South American invasion when Panama Isthmus closed. Most South American siskin species appeared close to Andean Mountains spine (Figure 18).

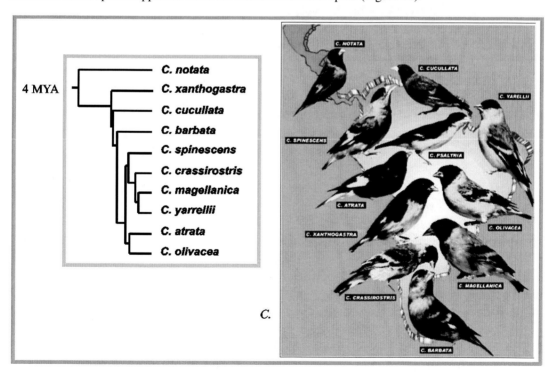

Figure 18. South American siskins. Note that *C. psaltria colombiana* is a North American bird belonging to the *C. tristis* radiation [10,30,31].

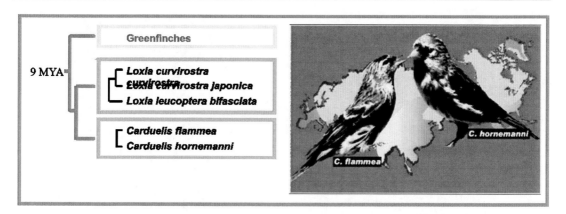

Figure 19. Linearized Neighbor Joining phylogeny of redpolls and crossbills [10,58].

Consideration should also be given to the possibility of classifying redpolls apart from the genus *Carduelis* and together with *Loxia*, since redpolls are genetically distant from the twite/linnet couple [10,58]. Previously, twite, linnet, and redpolls were considered as a subgroup (or even another genus, *Acanthis*) [11,50] within the genus *Carduelis*. The fact that genus *Loxia* and redpolls do not go together in [25] calculations is due to a distortion artifact caused by the *C. carduelis* group.

2. Genus Serinus: Radiations Intermingled in Time with those of Genus Carduelis

Genus *Serinus* species (canaries) occur in Palearctic and Afro-tropical areas. They are included within the *Carduelini* tribe, and comprise thirty-two to forty-five [3] different species. They usually thrive in Africa and some species also inhabit central and southern Europe, Turkey, Middle East and Arabia [11]. Most of them are small or slender finches, generally green, greenish-yellow, brown or grey with dark streaks, usually with distinctly bright rump patch and forked or notched tail [11]. Canaries' monophyly has been questioned on the basis of behavior and life history traits [3]. Species classification based on morphology, as well as on biogeographic distribution patterns [3] recognized five monophyletic groups: *Serinus sensu stricto* (*S. alario*, *S. citrinella*, *S. canicollis*, *S. syriacus*, *S. pusillus*), *Poliospiza* (*S. leucopterus*, *S. striolatus*, *S. gularis*, *S. tristriata*), *Dendrospiza* (*S. citrinelloides*, *S. hyposticta*, *S. scotops*), *Crithagra* (*S. flaviventris*, *S. sulphuratus*, *S. donaldsoni*, *S. albogularis*), *Ochrospiza* (*S. leucopygius*, *S. reichenowi*, *S. atrogularis*, *S. citrinipectus*, *S. mozambicus*, *S. dorsostriatus*, *S. xanthopygius*). The molecular phylogeny obtained by us [17] was to a great extent coincidental with these phenotypically defined groups with the exception of *Serinus citrinella* (citril finch, Figure 12); also, African canaries were classified in a simpler way (Figure 21) [17].

Most canaries are beautifully colored, widespread, and familiar to bird watchers and other people [3,11,50].

The relationships of the species within the genus *Serinus* and to other *Carduelini* finches have not been fully resolved [3,9,73], particularly regarding Old World species [72]. Parallel evolution of many characters seems to be an obstacle to phylogenetic resolution (for review, see [9,31]).

It is also intriguing that the *Serinus* species are mostly confined to Africa and the Mediterranean Basin; however, it is believed that their ancestors came from the Palearctic region (probably from somewhere around the Europe/Asia junctions [11]). Notwithstanding, two species, *S. thibetanus*, which exists in Central Asia, and *S. estherae*, which lives in parts of the Malay Archipelago, are relict species isolated from the Mediterranean-African area [11,17]. *Serinus syriacus* was included in the Eurasian-African canaries [31], *Serinus totta* was a small Afican canary [25,31], and *Linurgus olivaceus* another basal canary [25].

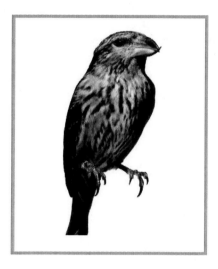

Figure 20. Common crossbill (*Loxia curvirostra*).

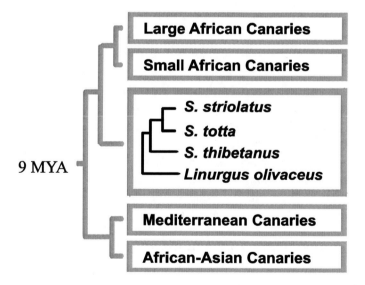

Figure 21. NJ phylogeny of genus *Serinus*, also confirmed by Maximum Likelihood and Bayesian Inference [17,25].

Although many scholars think that Pleistocene temperature variations (glaciations) and the subsequent isolation are the most important factors that provoke the appearance of new extant bird species [35,74], recent contradictory evidence exists which suggests that speciation of some genera and orders may have occurred long before [27,75-78], particularly in passerines [16] and in particular in *Carduelini* [9,10,13,17,25,72].

In order to estimate the tempo of evolution of *Serinus* species, the calculations done by Takahata, Grant, and Klein [5] to assess the time of appearance of Galapagos Darwin's finches were followed. A UPGMA dendrogram (Figure 21) was constructed because this type of phylogenetic tree is more suitable for estimating coalescence time than other methods [79]. Its topology was fully confirmed by bootstrap values and other tree construction methodologies (Parsimony, Neighbor Joining, and Maximum Likelihood) [17,25,31]. Next, a time scale for the UPGMA tree was obtained by comparing the cytochrome b DNA sequences of the pheasant [80] and the chicken [7], two species that are believed to have diverged around 19 MYA [6]. The per-lineage comparison yields an overall evolutionary rate of $3.97 \times 10^{-9} \pm 0.37$. This substitution rate is approximately 0.4% per MYA, which represents a surprisingly fast radiation for Serinus species (also suggested for *Carduelis* by Fehrer [9]). Other documented songbird radiations include the following: genus *Zonotrichia* has a 4.1% rate of nucleotide substitution, but for only seven species, and genus *Pipilo* has a substitution rate of 6.4% for only six species [28,29]. However, substitution rate for cranes' evolutionary groups is similar [8].

It is remarkable that the average percent of nucleotide divergence obtained among the 20 *Serinus* species is only 4%. This value represents a surprisingly fast radiation for *Serinus* species (also suggested for *Fringillinae* by Fehrer [9]). This molecular clock calibration may be correct because first, fossil data are included in the estimation of the species divergence time; this was considered accurate by Takahata, Klein, and Grant [5]). It is a clear advantage since the bird fossil record is fragmentary, particularly for small birds like *Serinus*. A node groups together canaries from the Mediterranean area and certain canaries from South Africa, Central Africa, and Asia (Figure 21).

Although different *Serinus* groups are in general concordantly placed in dendrograms obtained by using parsimony, NJ, ML, Bayesian, and UPGMA [2,17,25,31], some bootstrap values for nodes joining a few species belonging to otherwise well-established (high bootstrap) groups are low; this may reflect that not all extant species are tested. It may not be the case for the *Serinus* species, since only species phenotypically related and geographically close to the tested ones are missing from the study [3,11]. In addition, parental species are extinct and/or each group of bootstrap-supported nodes represents radiations of separate subfamilies; furthermore, the species (and thus DNA) are too similar and have appeared within a relatively short time span. The latter two may be more favored hypotheses, and although more studies are necessary to support them, other close *Fringillidae* genera are definitively outgroups (these include several ones that already existed in the early Miocene epoch: *Passer*, *Lagonostica*, *Lonchura*, *Pyrrhula*, *Rhodopechys*, and *Carpodacus* [17,58]. In general, established clades within dendrograms are geographically related.

Both parsimony and NJ trees [17] basically established the same groups for genus *Serinus*. The grouping within the genus may be as follows (distribution range shown in photographs has been taken from Clement, Harris, and Davies [11].

- Small African Canaries
- Large African canaries
- Mediterranean Canaries
- African-Asian medium-sized canaries, including the black-headed canary, yellow-crowned canary, and red-fronted serin —possibly related to Mediterranean canaries

and once sharing or connected by Saharan habitat), which now exist in fragmented habitats (juvenile red-fronted serins (Asia) and black-headed canaries (South Africa) are almost identical [17]—.

- Other Canaries: Oriole Finch (*Linurgus olivaceus*) and other relict Canaries (*S. totta*, *S. striolatus*, and *S. thibetanus*)
- Small African Canaries: Yellow-rumped Seedeater (*S. atrogularis*), White-rumped Seedeater (*S. leucopygius*), Lemon-breasted Seedeater (*S. citrinipectus*), White-bellied Canary (*S. dorsostriatus*), African Citril (*S. citrinelloides*), Yellow-fronted Canary (*S. mozambicus*), Cape Siskin (*S. totta*)

Big and small African canaries had already been distinguished as different clades by using phenotype characters [9,81], but they are not generally coincidental with our own data groups [17,25,31].

The small ones (10–13 cm) have a varied, powerful, and very nice singing, particularly the small and modestly gray-colored *S. leucopygius* (African singer; Figure 22). This contrasts with other big African canaries (15–16 cm; Figure 23), whose singing is more monotonous and not so varied and powerful. They cluster together in Parsimony, NJ, ML, Bayesian, and UPGMA dendrograms, with different bootstrap values [17,25,31].

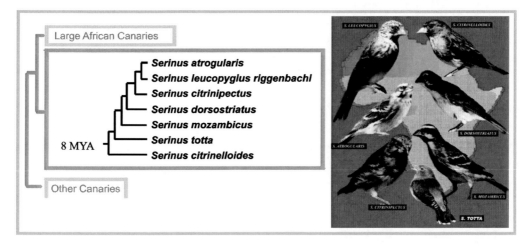

Figure 22. Small African Canaries [17,25,31].

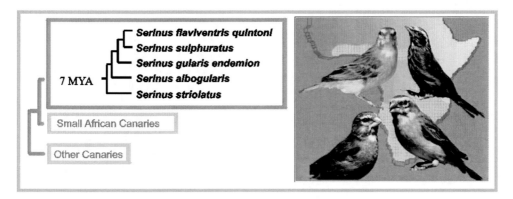

Figure 23. Large African Canaries [17,25,31].

Large African Canaries: Yellow Canary (*S. Flaviventris*), Brimstone Canary (*S. Sulphuratus*), Streaky-Headed Seedeater (*S. Gularis*), White-Throated Canary (*S. Albogularis*)

Large African canaries are all present in the extreme south of Africa (and also in Central Africa areas), while the small ones are more concentrated around the tropics; these size differences according to latitude are found in many species [35]. It is doubtful that big and small African *Serinus* finches have shared very close ancestors; if this is not so, the low bootstrap values linking small and big canaries may only reflect the lack of analysis of certain extant or extinct species. Relatedness of big and small African canaries with Mediterranean canaries may be relatively distant, since male hybrids obtained by crossing *S. canaria* with *S. sulphuratus*, *S. atrogularis*, and *S. mozambicus* are sterile [82]. However, male hybrid sterility may not be a sign of unrelatedness since F1 males from *S. canaria* and some South American siskins (i.e., *C. cucullata* and *C. xanthogaster*) are fertile [82]. This suggests that geographically closer species may develop hybridization barriers in the speciation process at meiotic, gamete, maturation, or other levels. The UPGMA dendrogram further splits small African canaries and places *S. citrinelloides* and *S. mozambicus* with the Mediterranean canaries (they did not show high bootstrap values in parsimony and/or NJ trees [17]); thus, a link between the two latter species may not be discarded even if sterile F1 males are obtained from *S. canaria* x *S. mozambicus* crosses [82].

In addition, the time of appearance calculation for African big canary species (Figure 23) [17,25,31] supports the hypothesis that vertebrate speciation also took place before Pleistocene glaciations in the American [10] and African Southern hemispheres, not only in North America [16].

African-Asian Canaries: Black-Headed Canary (*S. Alario*), Cape Canary (*S. Canicollis*), Fire-Fronted Serin (*S. Pusillus*), Syrian Finch (*S. Syriacus*) [31]

Mediterranean canaries are probably linked to certain African and Asian *Serinus* birds by common and extinct ancestors (Figure 24). They are strikingly dissimilar in color and general phenotype. However, chicks of *S. alario* and *S. syriacus* (Middle East) are almost identical in shape and color (Arnaiz-Villena A, personal observation). The case of *S. alario* is a typical adaptation to nesting close to earth and not in green trees: green has disappeared for black and white [17].

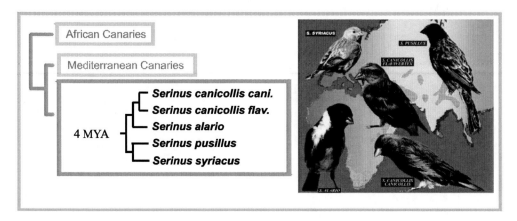

Figure 24. Afro-asiatic canaries [17,25,31].

Therefore, maintaining the name *Alario alario* instead of *Serinus alario* is not justified. This may be a reflection on how climate changes during the last 7 MYA, when the ancestors of this group may have already existed [17], and a relative isolation thereafter have caused drastic changes in color and bill shape [35]. Otherwise, random drift would be another explanation to the phenotypic changes observed. The oldest species is probably *S. pusillus* (Asian) (Figure 24), and this group (and the whole genus *Serinus* [11]) may be Asiatic in origin. In particular, the very recent Sahara desiccation which occurred about 10,000 years ago [83] may have helped to separate the original Northwestern and Northeastern African members of the group.

Mediterranean Canaries: Wild and Domestic Island Canary (*S. Canaria*), European Serin (*S. Serinus*)

Canaries from the Mediterranean area (Figure 25) comprise two species: serin and the wild canary from the Canary Islands; the caged domestic canary was bred in captivity for the first time about 500 years ago (when Europeans invaded the Islands) and was thus separated from the wild species. Also, the closest living relative to the wild canary is the Mediterranean serin, confirming the expectations [3,11] based on phenotypes, on fertile male hybrids and 20% female hybrids, and on geography [35]. Otherwise, random drift would be another explanation to the phenotypic changes observed.

Other Canaries: Oriole Finch (*Linurgus Olivaceus*) and Other Relict *Serinus* (*S. Totta, S. Thibetanus, S. Striolatus*) [17,25,31]

Our trees put together two species that are very different in size (*S. striolatus*, 15 cm; *S. thibetanus*, 11 cm) and plumage (Figure 26); they are not related taxa according to the low bootstrap values obtained. They may be the most ancient extant canaries and may also be relicts of primeval canaries. Both lineages (and, in this case, species) seem to come from 9 MYA (Miocene). *Serinus striolatus* may have become confined to Africa from a wider and also Asiatic range after climate changes occurred in the Middle East because of the Red Sea opening (10–5 MYA) and/or because of more recent glaciations [32].

Serinus thibetanus may have become isolated after Himalayan and Alpine orogenesis (5 MYA). Both of them, according to our molecular data [10], are included within the genus *Serinus* and not within *Carduelis*, as some authors have proposed [11], and show that Miocene speciation also occurred in Eurasia.

The Bayesian analysis place *Linurgus olivaceus* within subfamily *Fringillinae* when compared to members of most of the families and subfamilies of songbirds (Figure 9) [3,25,30], which is concordant with Sibley's bird classification [3]. It was found to belong to tribe *Carduelini*, and it is integrated within a strongly supported group that clusters all the species from genera *Serinus*, *Carduelis* and *Loxia*, appearing in a single branch as a basal species close to African canaries. No sister taxa have been found, most likely due to the lack of extinct species in the analyses [17,25,30,31].

Serinus totta seems to be the oldest of the small African canary group (Figure 22) [25,31].

According to our results [10,17,25,30,31], the speciation of canaries and goldfinches started in the Miocene Epoch, about 9 – 10 MYA. The oriole finch is basal to many *Carduelis* and *Serinus* species (Figure 9a); thus, *Linurgus'* ancestor may or may not be the ancestor of some extant canaries and goldfinches-siskins, but it is certain that it belongs to the same polyphyletic group of radiations, which started in the late Miocene (23 – 25 MYA), since comparision with all other *Passeriformes* has been done.

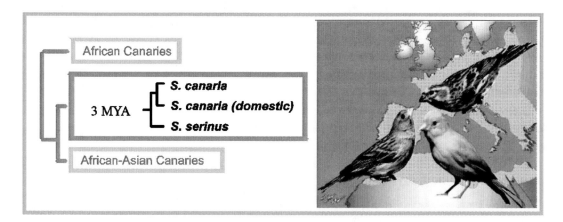

Figure 25. Mediterranean Canaries [17,25,31].

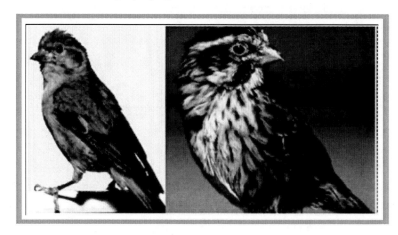

Figure 26. Relict canaries *S. thibetanus* (left) and *S. striolatus* (right) [17].

Convergent Evolution

We already saw a case in *Estrildinae* finches, between red-browed firetail, *Neochmia temporalis* and common waxbill, *Estrilda astrild* (Figure 7) [22]. In this case, convergent evolution towards black head and dark green colors is clearly found between both genetically unrelated oriole finch (*Linurgus olivaceus*) and Antillean siskin (*Carduelis dominicensis*, Figure 27), the latter belonging to the *Carduelis pinus* radiation [30]. This is most probably due to the fact that these two birds live in humid forests and a dark color (conferred by changes in carotenoid and melanin metabolism) [35].

On the other hand, the Bayesian phylogenetic analysis shows that phenotypically distinct birds are indeed genetically close [10,25]. Some examples have been reported here (Figures 7, 11, 12, 13, 29, 32).

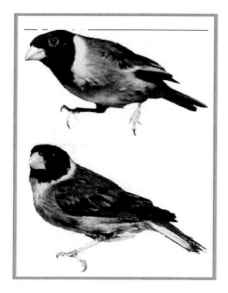

Figure 27. Convergent evolution in *L. olivaceus* (up) and *C. dominicensis* (down) [25,31].

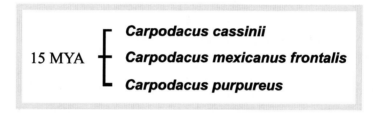

Figure 28. American "*Carpodacus*" [25,59].

3. Sheading Different and Split Rosefinches (genus carpodacus) Radiations

At this time of knowledge, "rosefinch" is a misleading name based on a vague color common character (some birds are red and some almost lack pink color), and since genus *Carpodacus* has been split in several genetic-evolutive groups according to phylogenetic NJ and Bayesian tree [25,58] (Figure 10), we will refer to "*Carpodacus*" birds until a clearer classification is established. They thrive in America, Asia, and one species in Africa (*Carpodacus syriacus* in Sinai Peninsula), and another one in Europe (*Carpodacus erythrinus*).

Altogether, four different "Carpodacus" finch evolutive radiations are described by us. If we take into account the "arid-zone" finches (Figure 32) [2,44], which group birds of three genera —*Carpodacus*, *Leucosticte*, and *Rhodopechys*—, five splits are found (see 'Arid-Zone Finches' on page 38).

American "Carpodacus" finches (C. mexicanus, C. cassinii)

Most "*Carpodacus*" finches are closer to the genus *Carduelis* than the other birds studied here. The head, beak, and body characteristics are more like those of a *Montifringilla* spp. than to many "*Carpodacus*" finches (unpublished results). *C. mexicanus* and *C. cassinii* form an altogether different evolutive radiation from Eurasian "*Carpodacus*" finches (Figure 28).

North American *Carpodacus purpureus* was also found to belong to this radiation (John Klicka, personal communication).

Haematospiza sipahi / Carpodacus erythrinus roseatus

The relatively large *Haematospiza sipahi* (18-19 cm, Figure 29) is included within the genus *Carpodacus*. *H. sipahi* is the one single member of genus *Haematospiza* [11], and has been related to *Coccothraustes coccothraustes* and *Eophona* [11]. This is not confirmed, and it is a bigger genetic sister species of a "*Carpodacus*" finch, *C. erythrinus roseatus* [25,58].

Uragus sibiricus / Carpodacus rubicilloides

The long-tailed "*Carpodacus*" finch (*Uragus sibiricus*), is definitively a sister species of *Carpodacus rubicilloides*. *U. sibiricus* was classified as the only species belonging to the genus *Uragus* because it has a "*Carpodacus*" body and a *Pyrrhula* beak; it is definitely a sister species of *Carpodacus rubicilloides* (Figure 29) [25,58]. *Uragus* may have changed its beak from that of *C. rubicilloides* (or its ancestor) as an adaptation to eat mainly buds, like *Pyrrhula*. This is another example of beak change in a relatively short time (Figure 29) [11,35,58].

The relationship of *U. sibiricus* with *Urocynchramus pylzowi* (pink-tailed rosefinch) should be studied in the future because of their phenotypic similarities and close geographical range (more limited for the latter, in central China); *Urocynchramus* may also belong to this genetic radiation [11,25,58].

Carpodacus pulcherrimus Radiation

Other "*Carpodacus*" finches are joined together, being *C. pulcherrimus* the oldest one [58]. In the following years, other Eurasian "*Carpodacus*" finches may be included with this one, or another hereby described radiation (Figures 28, 29). Four different evolutive radiations have been described by us, including American "*Carpodacus*" [25,58].

4. Grosbeak Radiation

This evolutive radiation appeared earlier than *Carduelis*, *Loxia*, *Carpodacus* and *Pyrrhula* radiations [58]. Their phenotypic and living uses of this group is detailed in [84].

Hawfinch (*C. coccothraustes*) is related to the bird groups stated in Figure 30, in particular with *Eophona* species, already considered by some investigators to be grosbeaks together with the hawfinch [11]). *C. coccothraustes* and *Eophona* species probably have close genetic relationship with the New World *Hesperiphona* species, and this should be studied; *C. coccothraustes* seems to be ancestral to *Eophona* species [25,58]. *Mycerobas* and *Eophona* birds are closely related, the latter being more ancient and possible the common ancestor to both genera.

The genera *Eophona* and *Mycerobas* are closely related in all trees with high statistical support. Whether they should be considered a single or two different genera is unclear, and the two missing Mycerobas species (*M. icteroides* and *M. melanozanthos*) should be tested in the future. The phenotypical relationship between *Mycerobas* and *Eophona* genera had been previously established [11].

Grosbeaks seem to have appeared on Earth earlier than the genera *Carduelis*, *Loxia*, *Carpodacus* and *Pyrrhula* in accordance with the hypothesized timing [58].

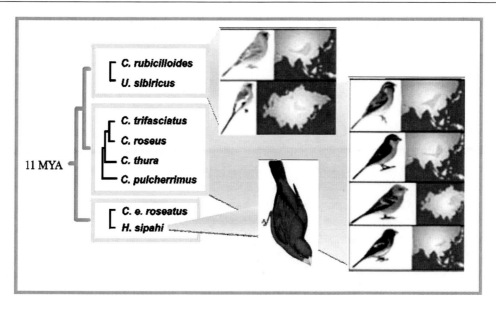

Figure 29. Eurasian "*Carpodacus*" [58].

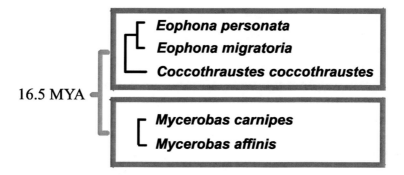

Figure 30. Grosbeaks [58].

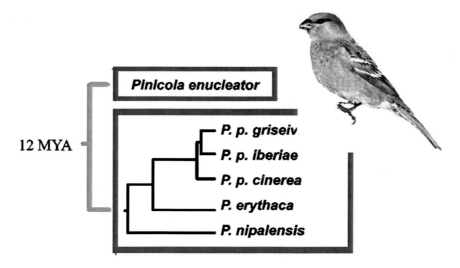

Figure 31. Bullfinches. Photography: *P. enucleator* [58].

5. Bullfinches (Genus Pyrrhula) and their Ancestor, the Pine Grosbeak (Pinicola enucleator)

These finches have a Palearctic distribution, including the Azores Islands and Japan. In the present chapter, we collected species and subspecies representing the entire geographic range. Their beak has evolved to eat buds [11]. The classification and phenotype is specified in [84].

Pine grosbeak (*Pinicola enucleator*, presently classified within genus *Pinicola*, 2 species, Figure 31) groups with bullfinches, and is probably one of the most ancient finches of the genus *Pyrrhula*, together with *Pyrrhula nipalensis*. Monophyly of this new group seems to be evident, since the statistical strength of the node is significantly high [2,58]. Therefore, *Pinicola* is not related to *Loxia* or *Carpodacus* as previously thought [11] and must share a common antecessor with bullfinches. Pine grosbeak would be the one *Pyrrhula* finch, found in North America; thus, *Pyrrhula* and *Pinicola* show a Holoarctic distribution. Pine grosbeak has been grouped with the red-headed rosefinch (*Pinicola subhimachala*) based on phenotypic characters in the genus *Pinicola* (only these 2 species). Both are larger (length ca. 22 cm) than *Pyrrhula* and *Carpodacus* finches. However, the genus Pinicola might be split between *Pyrrhula* (pine grosbeak) and *Carpodacus* (*C. subhimachala*, or red-headed rosefinch), the latter sharing many phenotypic characteristics with *Carpodacus* finches except for the much bigger size (length 20 cm). Size should not be a criterion for including the red-headed rosefinch within the genus *Carpodacus*, since the bigger *Haematospiza sipahi* (19 cm in length) is a sister species of *Carpodacus erythrinus roseatus* (Figure 29). The phenotypically defined subspecies *Pyrrhula pyr. cinerea* and *griseiventris* are concordant with the molecular subspecies status suggested here. The time of divergence of the *Pyrrhula* species (11 MYA) seems to be more recent than that of grosbeaks and "*Carpodacus*" finches but earlier than the crossbill-redpoll divergence time [58].

6. 'Arid-zone' Finches

A long lasting microgeographical study of *Fringillinae* birds by using mitochondrial DNA phylogenies has allowed us to define a group of monophyletic *Carpodacus / Rhodopechys / Leucosticte* birds, all of which thrive in arid areas [2,44]. This is in fact the fifth split of "*Carpodacus*" finches, based on evolutionary phylogenetics. This 'arid-zone' group is clearly separated from other *Carduelini* radiations according to maximum likelihood and Bayesian methodologies (Figures 9, 10) [2,44].

The Miocene Epoch is characterized by an initial cold peak, followed by a general Earth warming; the tundra was replaced by conifer woods in the corresponding areas between 17 and 14.5 million years ago (MYA) [23] when the temperatures were 6 °C higher than at present times [23]. However, after 14.5 MYA the temperatures started to drop and finally the Antarctica and Greenland became glaciated around 6 MYA. Simultaneously with this general cooling, vast arid regions appeared in Asia and Africa [23]. In addition, the Tibet plateau underwent its most important uplift during this cold Miocene period [23,85]. The heavy rain regime in the high Tibet-Himalayan peaks gave rise to the birth of deep and plentiful rivers (Ganges, Bramaputra, Yangtze and Mekong) which carry 25% of the total suspension materials that reach the oceans on Earth.

The ancestors of the new group of 'arid-zone' *Carduelini* might have appeared 13.5 MYA [44]. This is roughly coincidental with the appearance of vast arid areas in Africa and

Asia. This radiation might have started around this time in Asia (or less likely in Africa) from where some of the lineages later might have undergone dispersal during warmer conditions. This may be the case of *Leucosticte arctoa* now thriving both in Asia and America.

The arid-zone finches' plumage colors are not homogeneous and some *Leucosticte* and *Carpodacus* finches bear more melanin. This may suggest a more recent and disparate change in the respective 'arid-zone' finch environments.

More humid habitats (i.e., those of *Leucosticte* and *Carpodacus nipalensis* in comparison with *Rhodopechys* habitats) favor melanin dyed feathers, because it protects plumage from bacterial degradation by humidity [46]. Carotenoids, the other major pigments responsible for plumage coloration [35], are scarce in dry areas, but *Carpodacus nipalensis* also feeds on berries at high altitudes [11] and this may cause the intense male purple face coloring at breeding.

Also, *C. nipalensis* has the darkest plumage colors among "*Carpodacus*" finches [2,11,58], resembling *Leucosticte* finches in this respect. *C. nipalensis* was an outlier from "*Carpodacus*" finches [2,11].

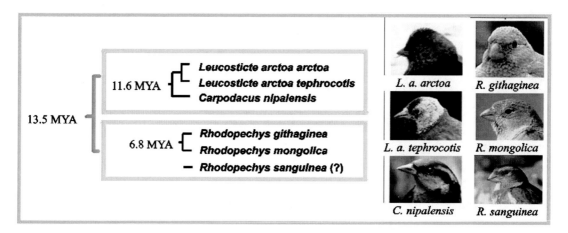

Figure 32. 'Arid-Zone' Finches [2].

7. Non-extant genus rhodopechys

In summary, according to our phylogenetic analyses based on mitochondrial cytochrome b DNA sequences, the genera *Rhodopechys* and *Carpodacus* should be revised because this 'arid-zone' separate evolutionary group comprises species belonging to both of the genera. Further analyses using nuclear and other markers could be required to complete the phylogenetic findings presented in this chapter, and a taxonomical revision of these genera is needed since only monophyletic clades should be used in a biological systematics, not only with the species studied here [3,58].

Finally, genus *Rhodopechys* would comprise *R. / Bucanetes githaginea* and, perhaps (not tested), *R. sanguinea*, although the later is geographically and phenotypically close to *R. mongolica* (Figure 32).

Rhodopechys obsoleta has already been included in the greenfinch radiation (Figures 13, 14) [44].

CONCLUSION

Our genetic studies on *Passerinae* birds' genetics and evolutionary radiations lead us to the following conclusions [3,12]:

1. Genus *Passer* (Old World Sparrows)

a) These birds probably originated in Africa, being *Passer melanurus* the extant most ancient ancestor.

b) This genus is not related to *Ploceus*, and to New and Old World *Emberizinae*.

c) Genus *Petronia* is a possible ancestral and closest group.

d) *Passer hispaniolensis italiae* seems a subspecies of *Passer domesticus* (grey-headed Old World sparrow).

2. *Estrildinae* Finches

a) This genetically well defined family neatly separates from *Vidua* species and includes several evolutive radiations in Africa, southern Asia (Indic Ocean), Indic and Pacific Ocean Islands, and Australia.

b) There is a clear convergent evolution of African common waxbill (*Estrilda astrild*) and Australian red-browed firetail (*Neochmia temporalis*). They both have a similar face and red eyebrows and a distant genetic relationship.

c) Each evolutive radiation is not confined or separated by geographical barriers; radiations exist which include different species throughout the range (i.e.: Africa + Asia + Indic and Pacific Ocean isdlands + Australia).

d) It is suggested that this radiation may have originated in India when Indian Plate induced a vigorous Tibet Plateau uplift (25 MYA), which set up present monsoon rainfall regime. A mixed Indian-Australian-African basal radiation has been defined — (African silverbill (*Lonchura cantans*), Indian silverbill (*Lonchura malabarica*), and Australian diamond firetail (*Stagonopleura guttata*).

3. Tribe *Cardinalini*

a) Grosbeaks (genera *Coccothraustes*, *Eophona* and *Mycerobas*) are genetically similar, being *Coccothraustes* an *Eophona* genus' ancestor. New World Hesperiphona species may be related to Old World grosbeaks.

4. Tribe *Carduelini*

a) Previous genus *Carpodacus* species have been named '"*Carpodacus*" finches', and the genus has been split in five different genera evolutionary groups.

b) American "*Carpodacus*" finches form a separate evolutive radiation. House finch (*C. mexicanus*) and Cassinii's finch (*C. cassinii*) and purple finch (*C. purpureus*) are included in this group.

c) Scarlet finch (*Haematospiza sipahi*), the single species of genus *Haematospiza*, is genetically a sister of Hodgson's "*Carpodacus*" finch (*C. erythrinus roseatus*). Other *Carpodacus erythrinus* finches (and others) may also belong to this radiation.

d) Long-tailed rosefinch (*Uragus sibiricus*), the single species of genus *Uragus*, is closely related to the much bigger eastern great "*Carpodacus*" finch (*C. rubicilloides*, 19 cm). This represents again a single evolutionary radiation in which "*Carpodacus*" or other finches may be added in the future.

e) Beautiful "*Carpodacus*" finch (*C. pulcherrimus*) is apparently the oldest species of a group of "*Carpodacus*" finches. More non tested species are likely to be joined this radiation (Figure 30)

f) Dark rosefinch (*Carpodacus nipalensis*) is outgroup of the "*Carpodacus*" finches group, and clusters together with rosy mountain finch in phylogenetic dendrograms (Asian *Leucosticte arctoa arctoa* and North American *Leucosticte arctoa tephrocotis*), trumpeter finch (*Rhodopechys / Bucanetes githaginea*), and Mongolian finch (*Rhodopechys mongolica*). We have named all these "arid-zone birds", because of their cold or hot arid habitats. More *Leucosticte* subspecies will probably join this group. Crimson-winged finch (*Rhodopechys sanguinea*) could also be included.

g) Genus *Rhodopechys* needs to be revised since desert finch (*R. obsoleta*) is a greenfinch, probably the extant ancestral form. It may have to be removed from taxonomical works.

h) Pine grosbeak (*Pinicola enucleator*) is one of the two species of genus *Pinicola*, but it clusters together with bullfinches (genus *Pyrrhula*) as an ancestor. The suggested affinities of genus *Pinicola* with *Carpodacus* and *Loxia* [11] do not genetically exist. It is likely that red-headed rosefinch (*Pinicola subhimachala*), the second Pinicola species, also belongs in this *P. enucleator / Pyrrhula* radiation, or otherwise to a "*Carpodacus*" finches radiation.

Genus Carduelis (Goldfinches and Siskins)

a) Several parallel-in-time evolutive radiations have been observed starting around middle Miocene Epoch.

b) Citril finch (*C. citrinella*, formerly *Serinus citrinella*) [12] is an evolutive radiation, together with Eurasian goldfinch (*C. carduelis*). Citril finch subspecies from Corsica and Sardinia was probably European goldfinch's ancestor.

c) Crossbills (genus *Loxia*) and redpolls (*C. flammea* and *C. hornemanni*) belong to a single evolutive group. Genus *Loxia* could be included within genus *Carduelis*.

d) Twite (*C. flavirostris*) and linnet (*C. cannabina*) may be a single evolutive radiation. Thus, postulated genus *Acanthis* (twite, linnet and redpolls) does not exist. On the other hand, twite and linnet might have a genetic relationship with North American *C. tristis* radiation.

e) Three different North American siskin radiations have occurred.

1. Eurasian siskin (*C. spinus*) has given rise to pine siskin (*C. pinus, C. pinus perplexus*), Antillean siskin (*C. dominicensis*), and black-capped siskin (*C. atriceps*).

2. The second North American goldfinch radiation comprises Lawrence's goldfinch (*C. lawrencei*), dark-backed goldfinch —*C. psaltria hesperophilus* (western USA, no black, but green back), *C. psaltria psaltria* (varied degree of black on back), and *C. psaltria colombiana* (very dark back , range extending through Central to South American Andes down to northern Peru)—. The ancestor of this group which most likely linked it with *C. spinus* has disappeared —Major Histocompatibility Complex (MHC) data, unpublished—.

3. Black-headed siskin (*C. notata*) from the Mexican mountains has given rise to the South American radiation of siskins. This happened after 3 MYA when Panama Isthmus closed and mesothermal plants, appropriate for siskin feeding, passed to the Andean Spine. *C. notata*'s link to C. spinus is also missing, but MHC data links *C. notata* with *C. spinus* and South American siskins, particularly with black siskin (*C. atrata*, unpublished).

f) Greenfinches are one of the earliest *Carduelis* radiations. Its ancestor is desert finch (*Rhodopechys obsoleta*), which may now be called *Carduelis obsoleta*, if nomenclature committees decide to change it.

Genus Serinus (Canaries). Several Clades have been Observed:

a) Mediterranean Canaries. Canary (*S. canaria*) from Canary and Atlantic Islands is the origin of all pet-shop canaries. It is also the origin of the red canary, the first genetically engineered animal (Bremen, 1913). It forms an evolutive radiation with serin (*S. serinus*).

b) Big African canaries. The earliest is the streaky-headed seedeater (*S. gularis*). This group has several heavily built canaries with a poor singing.

c) Small African canaries. White-bellied canary (*S. dorsostriatus*) is apparently the oldest species of this radiation, which also comprises yellow-rumped seedeater (*S. atrogularis*), white-rumped seedeater (*S. leucopygius*), lemon-breasted seedeater (*S. citrinipectus*), African citril (*S. citrinelloides*), and yellow-fronted canary (*S. mozambicus*) and Cape siskin (*S. totta*).

d) African-Eurasian canaries. Red-fronted serin (*S. pusillus*) earliest appeared in this group, which also comprises black-headed canary (*S. alario*), Cape canary (*S. canicollis*), and Syrian serin (*Serinus syriacus*).

e) Tibetan siskin (*S. thibetanus*) is a small, ancient, relict canary confined to Himalayan areas. It is clearly a *Serinus* with some *Carduelis* phenotypic characters.

f) Streaky seedeater (*S. striolatus*) is a relict canary confined to East Africa.

g) Cape siskin (*S. totta*) is a basal canary, and seems to be one of the oldest. In some phylogenies, it is linked to the small canary group, as a basal one.

h) Oriole finch (*Linurgus olivaceus*) is a basal canary, and probably one of the most ancient ones.

ACKNOWLEDGMENTS

This work was supported in part by grants from the Spanish Ministry of Health (FISS PI051039 and PI080838), Spanish Ministry of Foreign Affairs (A/9134/07 and A/17727/08) and three different *Mutua Madrileña Automovilista* grants.

REFERENCES

Allende, LM; Rubio, I; Ruiz-del-Valle, V; et al. The Old World sparrows (genus *Passer*) phylogeography and their relative abundance of nuclear mtDNA pseudogenes. *J.Mol.Evol.*, 2001, 53, 144-154.

Armani, GC. Guide des Passereaux Granivores. Paris: Delchaux and Niestle (ed), 1983.

Arnaiz-Villena, A, Ruiz-del-Valle, V; Reguera, R; Gomez-Prieto, P; Serrano-Vela, JI. What might have been the ancestor of New World siskins? *Open Ornithology Journal*, 2008, 1, 46-47.

Arnaiz-Villena, A; Alvarez-Tejado, M; Ruiz-del-Valle, V; et al. Phylogeny and rapid northern and southern hemisphere speciation of goldfinches during the Miocene and Pliocene epochs. *Cell.Mol.Life.Sci.*, 1998, 54, 1031-1041.

Arnaiz-Villena, A; Alvarez-Tejado, M; Ruiz-del-Valle, V; et al. Rapid radiation of canaries (Genus *Serinus*). *Mol.Biol.Evol.*, 1999, 16, 2-11.

Arnaiz-Villena, A; Gomez-Prieto, P; Reguera, R; Parga-Lozano, C. Estrildinae Finches from Africa, South Asia and Australia. *Open Ornithology Journal*, 2009, 2.

Arnaiz-Villena, A; Guillen, J; Ruiz-del-Valle, V; et al. Phylogeography of crossbills, bullfinches, grosbeaks, and rosefinches. *Cell.Mol.Life.Sci.*, 2001, 58, 1159-1166.

Arnaiz-Villena, A; Moscoso, J; Ruiz-del-Valle, V; et al. Bayesian phylogeny of *Fringillinae* birds: status of the singular African Oriole Finch (*Linurgus olivaceus*) and evolution and heterogeneity of genus *Carpodacus*. Acta Zoologica Sinica, 2007, 53, 826-834.

Arnaiz-Villena, A; Moscoso, J; Ruiz-del-Valle, V; et al. Mitochondrial DNA Phylogenetic Definition of a Group of 'Arid-Zone' Carduelini Finches. *Open Ornithology Journal*, 2008, 1, 1-7.

Arnaiz-Villena, A; Ruiz-del-Valle, V; Moscoso, J; Serrano-Vela, JI; Zamora, J. mtDNA phylogeny of North American *Carduelis pinus group*. *Ardeola*, 2007, 54, 1-14.

Arnaiz-Villena, A; Ruiz-del-Valle, V; Reguera, R; Gomez-Prieto, P; Serrano-Vela, JI. What might have been the ancestors of New World siskins? *Open Ornithology Journal*, 2008, 1, 46-47.

Avibase. Avibase http://avibase.bsc-eoc.org/avibase.jsp?lang=EN&pg=home

Avise, JC; Walker, D. Pleistocene phylogeographic effects on avian populations and the speciation process. *Proc.R.Soc.Lond B Biol.Sci.*, 1998, 265, 457-463.

Ball, S. Evolution, explanation, and the fact/value distinction. *Biology and Philosophy*, 1988, 3, 317-348.

Baseggio, G. Ibridologia (I). *Mondo degli Ucceli*, Bologna, Italy: 1995.

Bernis, F. An Ecological view of Spanish Avifaune with reference to the Nordic and Alpine Birds. *Acta XI Congr.Int.Orn.*, 1954, 1, 423-427.

Bioinformatics and Molecular Evolution. Universidad de Vigo http://darwin.uvigo.es/

Birkhead, T. *The Red Canary: The Story of the First Genetically Engineered Animal*. London, UK, 2003.

Bond, J. Derivation of the Antillean Avifauna. *Proceedings of the Academy of Natural Sciences of Philadelphia*, 1963, 115, 79-98.

Bond, J. Origin of the Bird Fauna of the West Indies. *The Wilson Bulletin*, 1948, 60, 207-229.

Borras, A; Senar, JC. Opportunistic breeding of the Citril Finch *Serinus citrinella*. *J.Orn.*, 1991, 132, 285-289.

Brooke, M; Birkhead, T. The Cambridge Encyclopaedia of Ornithology. Cambridge, England: 1991.

Brown, JM; Lomolino, MV. *Biogeography*. Sunderland, MA (USA): Sinauer (ed), 2006.

Bryant HProc.BostonSoc.Nat.Hist., 1866, 11, 93-

Burtt, EHJ; Ichida, JM. Gloger's rule, feather-degrading bacteria, and color variation among Song Sparrows. *Condor*, 2004, 106, 681-686.

Chappuis, C. Origine et evolution des vocalisations de certains oiseaux de Corse et des Baleares. Alauda 1976;

Chiappe, LM. The first 85 million years of avian evolution. *Nature*, 1995, 378, 349-355.

Chung, SL; Lo, CH; Zhang, Y; et al. Diachronous uplift of the Tibetan plateau starting 40Myr ago. *Nature*, 1998, 394, 769-773.

Clement, P; Harris, P; Davies, J. *Finches and Sparrows*. London, 1993.

Cox, B; Moore, P. *Biogeography: an ecological and evolutionary approach*. 6, illustrated ed. 2000.

Cox, R; Lowe, D. A conceptual review of regional-scale controls on the composition of clastic sediment and the co-evolution of continental blocks and their sedimentary cover. *Journal of Sedimentary Research*, 1995, 65, 1-12.

Cramp, S; Perrins, CM. *Handbook of the Birds of Europe*, the Middle East and North Africa, vol VIII, Crows to Finches. Oxford (UK): 1994.

Desjardins, P; Morais, R. Sequence and gene organization of the chicken mitochondrial genome. A novel gene order in higher vertebrates. *J.Mol.Biol.*, 1990, 212, 599-634.

Dickinson, EC; Pearson, D; Remsen, V; Roselaar, K; Schodde, R. *The Howard and Moore complete check list of the birds of the world*. 3rd ed. London: Dickinson EC (ed), 2003.

Edwards, AW. Assessing molecular phylogenies. *Science*, 1995, 267, 253-256.

Erard, C; Etchecopar, R. Contribution à l'étude des oiseaux d'Iran: résultats de la mission etchecopar, 1967. Paris, France: Editions du Muséum (ed), 1970.

Feduccia, A. Explosive Evolution in Tertiary Birds and Mammals. *Science*, 1995, 267.

Fehrer, J. Conflicting character distribution within different data sets on cardueline finches: artifact or history? *Mol.Biol.Evol.*, 1996, 13, 7-20.

Fehrer, J. Interspecies-Kreuzungen bei cardueliden Finken und Prachtfinken. Typen des lebens. Berlin, Pascal, 1993, 197-216

Felsenstein, J. *Confidence limits of phylogenies: an approach using the bootstrap. Evolution*, 1985, 39, 783-795.

Felsenstein, J. Evolutionary trees from DNA sequences: a maximum likelihood approach. *J.Mol.Evol.*, 1981, 17, 368-376.

Felsenstein, J. *Inferring phylogenies*, 2004.

Filardi, CE; Moyle, RG. Single origin of a pan-Pacific bird group and upstream colonization of Australasia. *Nature*, 2005, 438, 216-219.

Fleischer, RC; McIntosh, C; Tarr, CL. Evolution on a volcanic conveyor belt: using phylogeographic reconstructions and K-A-based ages of the Hawaiian Islands to estimate molecular evolutionary rates. *Mol.Ecol.*, 1998, 7, 533-545.

Gill, FB. *Ornithology*. New York, NY (USA): 2006.

Grant, P; Grant, R. Mating patterns of Darwin's Finch hybrids determined by song and morphology. *Biological Journal of the Linnean Society*, 1997, 60, 317-343.

Hackett, SJ. Molecular phylogenetics and biogeography of tanagers in the genus Ramphocelus (Aves). *Mol.Phylogenet.Evol.*, 1996, 5, 368-382.

Harlid, A; Janke, A; Arnason, U. The mtDNA sequence of the ostrich and the divergence between paleognathous and neognathous birds. *Mol.Biol.Evol.*, 1997, 14, 754-761.

Hasegawa, M; Thorne, JL; Kishino, H. Time scale of eutherian evolution estimated without assuming a constant rate of molecular evolution. *Genes Genet.Syst.*, 2003, 78, 267-283.

Hedges, SB; Parker; PH; Sibley, CG; Kumar, S. Continental breakup and the ordinal diversification of birds and mammals. *Nature*, 1996, 381, 226-229.

Helm-Bychowski, KM; Wilson, AC. Rates of nuclear DNA evolution in pheasant-like birds: evidence from restriction maps. *Proc.Natl.Acad.Sci.*, U.S.A., 1986, 83, 688-692.

Hillis, DM; Huelsenbeck, JP; Cunningham, CW. Application and accuracy of molecular phylogenies. *Science*, 1994, 264, 671-677.

Howell, S, Webb, S. A guide to the birds of Mexico and Northern Central America. Oxford (UK): 1995.

Huelsenbeck, JP; Ronquist, F. MRBAYES: Bayesian inference of phylogeny. *Bioinformatics*, 2001, 17, 754-755.

James, F. Environmental Component of Morphological-Differentiation in Birds. *Science*, 1983, 221, 184-186.

Klicka, J; Zink, R. Pleistocene effects on North American songbird evolution. *Proc.R.Soc.Lond B*, 1999, 266, 695-700.

Klicka, J; Zink, R. The importance of recent ice ages in speciation: a failed paradigm. *Science*, 1997, 277, 1666-1669.

Kocher, TD; Thomas, WK; Meyer, A; et al. Dynamics of mitochondrial DNA evolution in animals: amplification and sequencing with conserved primers. *Proc.Natl.Acad.Sci.*, U.S.A., 1989, 86, 6196-6200.

Kornegay, JR; Kocher, TD; Williams, LA; Wilson, AC. Pathways of lysozyme evolution inferred from the sequences of cytochrome b in birds. *J.Mol.Evol.*, 1993, 37, 367-379.

Krajewski, C; King, DG. Molecular divergence and phylogeny: rates and patterns of cytochrome b evolution in cranes. *Mol.Biol.Evol.*, 1996, 13, 21-30.

Kroemer, G; Zoorob, R; Auffray, C. Structure and expression of a chicken MHC class I gene. *Immunogenetics*, 1990, 31, 405-409.

Kumar S; Tamura, K; Nei, M. MEGA3: Integrated software for Molecular Evolutionary Genetics Analysis and sequence alignment. Brief.Bioinform. 2004, 5: 150-163.

Kutzbach, J; Bonan, G; Foley, J; Harrison, SP. Vegetation and soil feedbacks on the response of the African monsoon to orbital forcing in the early to middle Holocene. *Nature*, 1996, 384, 623-626.

Lanyon, W. Revision and probable evolution of the Myarchus flycatchers of the West Indies. 1967.

Maldonado, A. Evolution of the Mediterranean basins ans a detailed reconstruction of the Cenozoic paleoceanography. Oxford: Margalef R (ed), 1985.

Marten, JA; Johnson, NK. Genetic relationships of North American cardueline finches. *Condor*, 1986, 88, 409-420.

Mayr, E; Sort, L; Club, N. *Species taxa of North American birds: a contribution to comparative systematics*, 1970.

McEvedy, C. *The Penguin Atlas of African History*. London, 1980.

Moritz, C. Defining 'evolutionary significant units' for conservation. *Trends.Ecol.Evol.*, 1994, 9, 373-375.

Nei, M. *Molecular Evolutionary Genetics*. New York, NY (USA): 1987.

Ottaviani, M. Monographie des fringilles (Fringillinae - Carduelini). Histoire naturel et photographies. Ingre (France), Editions Prin, 2009.

Owens, IP. Male-only care and classical polyandry in birds: phylogeny, ecology and sex differences in remating opportunities. *Philos.Trans.R.Soc.Lond B Biol.Sci.*, 2002, 357, 283-293.

Pasquet, E; Thibault, JC. Genetic differences among mainland and insular forms of the Citril Finch *Serinus citrinella*. *Ibis*, 1997, 139, 679-684.

Paturi, F. In Haremberg Komunikation (ed): Die Kronik der Erde. Dortmund, Deutschland, 1991, 284-496

Posada, D; Crandall, KA. MODELTEST: testing the model of DNA substitution. *Bioinformatics*, 1998, 14, 817-818.

Pregill, G; Olson, SL. Zoogeography of West Indian Vertebrates in Relation to Pleistocene Climatic Cycles. *Annual Review of Ecology and Systematics*, 1981, 12, 75-98.

Ronquist, F; Huelsenbeck, JP. MRBAYES 3: Bayesian phylogenetic inference under mixed models. *Bioinformatics*, 2003, 19, 1572-1574.

Saetre, GP; Borge, T; Lindell, J; et al. Speciation, introgressive hybridization and nonlinear rate of molecular evolution in flycatchers. *Mol Ecol.*, 2001, 10, 737-749.

Salvin, O. *Proceedings of the Scientific Meetings of the Zoological Society of London*. 1863, 190.

Sangster, G. Genetic distance as a test of species boundaries in the Citril Finch *Serinus citrinella*: a critique and taxonomic reinterpretation. *Ibis*, 2000, 142, 487-490.

Sanz, J. Los dinosaurios voladores: historia evolutiva de las aves primitivas. 1ª, 1ª reimpresión ed. Madrid, España: Ediciones Libertarias/Prodhufi (ed), 1999.

Sibley, CG; Ahlquist, J. *Phylogeny and classification of birds*. New Haven, Conn.: 1990.

Smith, D; Funnel, B. *Atlas of Mesozoic and Cenozoic Coastlines*. Illustrated ed. Cambridge: 2009.

Sorenson, MD; Balakrishnan, CN; Payne, RB. Clade-limited colonization in brood parasitic finches (*Vidua* spp.). *Syst.Biol.*, 2004, 53, 140-153.

Summers-Smith, J. The Sparrows. Calton, Stafforrshire, England: T AA Poyser Ltd (ed), 1988.

Swofford, D. PAUP (phylogenetic analysis using parsimony), Version 4.0b2. 1996, Illinois, USA. Ref Type: Patent

Takezaki, N; Rzhetsky, A; Nei, M. Phylogenetic test of the molecular clock and linearized trees. *Mol.Biol.Evol.*, 1995, 12, 823-833.

Thorne, JL; Kishino, H; Painter, IS. Estimating the rate of evolution of the rate of molecular evolution. *Mol.Biol.Evol.*, 1998, 15, 1647-1657.

Todd, W. A study of the neotropical finches of the genus Spinus. *Annals of the Carnegie Museum*, 1926.

Uriarte-Cantolla, A. *Historia del Clima de la Tierra*. Vitoria, 2003.

Van den Elzen, R. Systematics and distribution patterns of Afrotropical Canaries. *Boon.Zool.Monogr*, 2000, 46, 133-143.

Van den Elzen, R; Nemeschkal, HL. Radiation in African canaries (Carduelidae): a comparison of different classificatory approaches. *Acta Congr.Int.Ornithol.*, 1991, 20, 459-467.

van Rossen, AJ. *Bull.Brit.Ornith.Club*, 1938, 58, 134-134.

Van-der-Meij, MMA; de-Baker, MAG; Bout, RG. Phylogenetic relationships of finches and allies based on nuclear and mitochondrial DNA. *Mol.Phylogenet.Evol.*, 2005, 34, 97-105.

Vaurie, C. The birds of the palearctic fauna: a systematic reference (Order Passeriformes). London (UK): 1959.

Vincek, V; O´Huigin, C; Satta, Y; et al. How large was the founding population of Darwin´s finches? *Proc. R.Soc.Lond B*, 1997, 264, 111-118.

Wilson, A. The Natural History of the Birds of the United States: Illustrated with Plates Engraved and Colored from Original Drawings taken from Nature, 1810, 133.

Wittzell, H; von Schantz, T; Zoorob, R; Auffray, C. Molecular characterization of three Mhc class II B haplotypes in the ring-necked pheasant. *Immunogenetics*, 1994, *39*, 395-403.

Yang, Z. Estimating the pattern of nucleotide substitution. *J.Mol.Evol.*, 1994, 39, 105-111.

Zamora, J; Lowy, E; Ruiz-del-Valle, V; et al. *Rhodopechys obsoleta* (desert finch): a pale ancestor of greenfinches (*Carduelis* spp.) according to molecular phylogeny. *J.Ornithol.*, 2006, 147, 448-456.

Zamora, J; Moscoso, J; Ruiz-del-Valle, V; et al. Conjoint mitochondrial phylogenetic trees for canaries (*Serinus* spp.) and goldfinches (*Carduelis* spp.) show several specific polytomies. *Ardeola*, 2006, 53, 1-17.

Zink, R; Dittmann, DL; Rootes, WL. Mitochondrial DNA variation and the phylogeny of *Zonotrichia*. The Auk 1991, 108: 578-584.

Zink, RM; Dittman, DL. Evolution of brown towhees: mitochondrial DNA evidence. *The Condor*, 1991, 93, 98-105.

APPENDIX. METHODOLOGY

A. Field Work

Photographs were taken with a Nikon N-90 camera equipped with a Nikon 80-200 zoom objective and automatic flash by A. Arnaiz-Villena.

B. Sampling and Sequencing

Blood from living birds was drawn after photographing by cutting the nail of legs locally anaesthetized with lidocaine ointment. Blood was collected in EDTA at 4 °C and frozen until use [10].

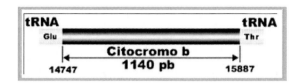

Figure 33. Cytochrome b gene.

DNA was obtained, and 924 bp of the mtDNA Cyt b gene was amplified with primers L14841 and H15767 as detailed in ref. 15. The BLAST program was used for sequence alignment (http://www.ncbi.nlm.nih.gov/BLAST).

The following calculations were carried out: number of substitutions (synonymous and non-synonymous), number of variable and phylogenetically informative sites, and the base composition according to codon position. **Saturation plots** were drawn to compare pairwise percent sequence divergence to pairwise transversion and pairwise transition divergence at first, second, and third codon positions [17].

C. Cyt-b

Phenotypic, behavioral and molecular evolution are not concordant [3]. At smaller divergences, mtDNA has been cited as a 'molecular clock', calibrated for vertebrates at an approximate divergence rate of 2% per MY [6,86]; however, an experimentally found mixed molecular / geological clock has been used here [10,17].

Since Kocher et al. [57], the mitochondrial cytochrome b gene (Figure 33) has been a popular source of DNA sequences for phylogenetic reconstruction, though few studies have considered the evolutionary dynamics of this gene and its encoded protein.

The power of DNA sequencing of Cyt b (or other orthologous genes) for solving taxonomy problems may be fully shown by analyzing as many as possible of the closest extant species, as was done in the present chapter. Relationships among very close species may, however, not be fully solved, as is observed in the case of South American siskins.

924 bp are sufficient to obtain an accurate phylogenetic tree (parsimony, NJ and UPGMA) in most cases [56] and overcome the uncertainties found in other songbird phylogenies by using only 307 bases of mt-Cyt b [9].

D. Phylogenetic Methods

Usually, several methods were combined. Two different estimates of percent divergence were used that serve as approximations of time since divergence: Kimura's (1980) two-parameter genetic distance and uncorrected pairwise divergence (p = N_d/n, where p is the percent sequence divergence, N_d is the number of nucleotides that differ between two sequences, and n is the total number of nucleotides compared [77,79]). The statistical significance of a particular sequence cluster was also evaluated by the confidence probability (CP) (CP = 1 − type [87]); this complements the bootstrap values.

Maximum parsimony (MP), NJ with maximum-likelihood distances, linearized NJ with Kimura biparametric distances and UPGMA with biparametric distance matrices were obtained with the PAUP*4.0b2 program, kindly provided by [88] and with the MEGA package program in the case of the linearized tree [89].

The trees were rooted with *Fringilla coelebs* or *Emberiza impetuani*. Sometimes, pheasant and chicken were used as a tree root [10,17].

1. Cladistic Methods

Maximum Parsimony Tree

The general idea of parsimony methods was given in their first mention in the scientific literature: Edwards and Cavalli-Sforza's (1963) declaration that the evolutionary tree is to be preferred that involves "the minimum net amount of evolution". We seek that phylogeny on which, when we reconstruct the evolutionary events leading to our data, there are as few events as possible. This raises two issues. First, we must be able to make a reconstruction of events, involving as few events as possible, for any proposed phylogeny. Second, we must be able to search among all possible phylogenies for the one or ones that minimize the number of events [90].

There are two methods of rooting a tree: the outgroup criterion and the use of a molecular clock.

For high change rates, we used **weighed parsimony**, which assigns a particular "weight", or phylogenetic importance, to each variable site.

2. Quantitative Methods

Unweighted Pair Group with Arithmetic Mean (UPGMA)

A Kimura biparametric distance matrix was used [10,87]. UPGMA methodology tends to perform poorly if the assumption of equal rate of Cyt b evolution among species does not reflect their actual evolution [56]. However, it seems to perform correctly in the closely related bird species used for this work since groups of taxa are similar to those obtained in NJ and parsimony dendrograms.

Neighbor Joining (NJ)

The UPGMA tree is not an exact method to infer phylogenies among species if a constant evolutionary rate does not occur, so we used other types of trees to validate the UPGMA tree topology [56]. Bootstrap values are calculated as a method of testing the topological robustness of trees calculated by parsimony and NJ methods [91], and low bootstrap branches are shown because the same tree branch is obtained by at least two different tree construction methods [92]. Also, the number of variable sites, including chicken, pheasant and chaffinch sequences (327 out of 924 Cyt b DNA bases) and phylogenetically informative sites (230) is sufficient to establish sound phylogenetic comparisons [56].

Maximum Likelihood (ML)

With this method, base composition and number of synonymous (dS) and non-synonymous (dN) distances are taken into account. For the ML analysis [93] we consider the following settings: two substitutions types; estimated transition / transversion ratio via ML; HKY85 model; empirical nucleotide frequencies; none assumed proportion of invariable sites and gamma distribution of rates at variable sites, divided in four categories as done by Yang [94] for mitochondrial DNA sequences.

Bearing in mind that variation of evolutionary rate among lineages may exist, we estimated the branch lengths by ML allowing rates to continuously change over time, according to the molecular clock model of Thorne et al. [95]. This model was successfully applied to several biological issues [96].

Bayesian Inference

For Bayesian tree analysis [97], program MrBayes 3.1.2 [98] is used. The model of evolution chosen is the one that most likely fit for the data set, according to program ModelTest 3.1 [99,100]; in this case, it was GTR+I+G, a general time reversible model that considers up to six different nucleotide substitution types, the proportion of invariable sites, and a gamma distribution of rates at variable sites, with the associated shape parameter 'alpha'. Two independent runs, with one cold chain and a number of heated chains depending on number of species, are performed along several million generations, sampling every 100 generations. The first 25% of samples are discarded. After that, both runs converge to a stationary distribution and the average standard deviation of split frequencies approaches zero. We only consider values under 0.01.

3. Linearized Trees

Linearized ML trees were constructed by assuming that evolutionary rates between lineages may be different [95]. PARAMCLOCK PAUP command was used for tree building. Divergence times were estimated assuming an evolutionary rate of 0.8% substitutions per site per MY, found by Fleischer et al. [101]. This rate is based on the Cyt b sequence divergence of Hawaiian honeycreepers, and external geological calibration points [44].

The time scale for the UPGMA tree was obtained by comparing mt Cyt b of chicken [102] and pheasant [103], two species that diverged 20 MYA [6] according to combined fossil and molecular comparison calculations. The comparison yields a value of 4% average amount of nucleotide substitution per lineage between the most distant *Carduelis* species arose in about 10 MY (Figure 9).

Times of species divergence are only a rough estimate. Standard error of the pheasant–chicken distance indicates that the calibration inaccuracy is about 10%. The chaffinch divergence time is closer to that inferred for chicken and pheasant than to divergence times inferred for *Carduelis*.

INDEX

J

K

L

M

N

O

P

R